MCQs
in Medical Microbiology
and Infectious Diseases

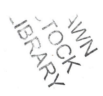

Other Examination Preparation Books Published by Petroc Press:

Balcombe	*Notes for the MRCP Part I*	1900603470
Bateson	*Basic Tests in Gastroenterology*	1900603772
Bateson	*MCQs in Clinical Gastroenterology*	1900603519
Bateson	*MCQs on the Upper Digestive Tract*	1900603373
Bateson & Stephen	*MCQs in Gastroenterology*	1900603403
Black & Kelleher	*MCQs in Anaesthesiology*	1900603454
Chakravorty	*Visual Aids to the MRCP Examination*	0792388739
Chong & Wong	*Survival Kit for MRCP Part II*	1900603063
Edgell	*Preparing for MRCP Part II Cardiology*	0792388690
Green	*More MCQs for Finals*	079238928X
Green (Ed.)	*The MRCPsych Study Manual:* 2nd edn	1900603527
Helmy & Mokbel	*EMQs for the PLAB*	1900603721
Hogston	*MCQs for the MRCoG Part II*	1900603551
Kazkaz *et al.*	*MCQs for the MRCP Part I*	1900603071
Kubba *et al.*	*MCQs for MFFP Part I*	1900603004
Levi	*Basic Notes in Psychiatry:* 2nd edn	1900603306
Levi	*Basic Notes in Psychotherapy*	1900603500
Levi	*Basic Notes in Psychopharmacology:* 2nd edn	1900603608
Levi	*MCQs in Psychiatry for MRCPsych*	1900603853
Levi	*PMPs for the MRCPsych Part II*	079238993X
Levi	*SAQs for the MRCPsych*	0746200994
Levy & Riordan Eva	*MCQs in Optics and Refraction*	1900603225
Levy & Riordan Eva	*MCQs for the FRCOphth*	1900603276
Levy & Riordan Eva	*MCQs for the MRCOphth*	1900603179
Mokbel	*MCQs in Applied Basic Medical Sciences*	1900603756
Mokbel	*MCQs in General Surgery*	1900603101
Mokbel	*MCQs in Neurology*	0792388577
Mokbel	*Operative Surgery and Surgical Topics for the FRCS/MRCS*	1900603705
Mokbel	*SAQs in Clinical Surgery-in-General for the FRCS*	190060390X
Ross & Emmanuel	*MCQs on Antimicrobial Therapy*	1900603411
Ross & Emmanuel	*MCQs in Medical Microbiology for MRCP*	0792388836
Ross & Emmanuel	*MCQs in Microbiology and Infection for FRCS*	1900603152
Rymer & Higham	*Preparing for the DRCoG*	1900603012
Sandler & Sandler	*MCQs in Cardiology for MRCP Pt I*	0792389999
Sandler & Sandler	*MCQs in Cardiology*	0792389387
Sandler & Sandler	*More MCQs in Cardiology for MRCP Pt I*	0792388402
Sikdar	*MCQs in Basic Sciences for MRCPsych Pt II*	190060356X

Obtainable from all good booksellers or, in case of difficulty, from Plymbridge Distributors Limited, Plymbridge House, Estover Road, PLYMOUTH, Devon, PL6 7PZ, Tel. 01752–202300, Fax 01752–202333.

MCQs
in
Medical Microbiology
and
Infectious Diseases

P. W. Ross TD, MD, FRCPath, FRCPE, CBiol, FIBiol, FLS
Reader in Medical Microbiology, University of Edinburgh
Honorary Consultant Bacteriologist, Royal Infirmary, Edinburgh
Examiner, Royal College of Pathologists and Royal College of Surgeons of
*   Edinburgh*
President, Scottish Microbiology Association

F. X. S. Emmanuel MB, BS, MSc, PhD, FRCPath
Consultant Bacteriologist, Royal Infirmary, Edinburgh
Honorary Senior Lecturer in Medical Microbiology, University of Edinburgh
Examiner, Royal College of Pathologists

with a Foreword by

A. M. Geddes CBE, MBChB, FRCP, FRCPE, FRCPath, FFPHM

THIRD EDITION

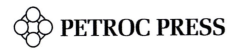 **PETROC PRESS**

Petroc Press, an imprint of LibraPharm Limited

Distributors
Plymbridge Distributors Limited, Plymbridge House, Estover Road, Plymouth PL6 7PZ, UK

First edition 1993 © Kluwer Academic Publishers
Reprinted 1995
Second edition 1997 © LibraPharm Limited
Third edition 2000
Reprinted 2001

Published by LibraPharm Limited
Gemini House
162 Craven Road
Newbury
Berkshire
RG14 5NR
UK

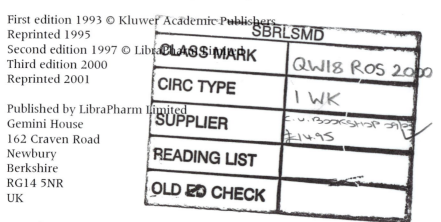

A catalogue record for this book is available from the British Library

ISBN 1 90060308 X

Typeset by Richard Powell Editorial and Production Services, Basingstoke, Hampshire RG22 4TX
Printed and bound in the United Kingdom by MWL Digital Solutions Ltd, Pontypool, Mon NP4 0DQ

Contents

Foreword

The ideal examination has not yet been devised. Essay questions require a degree of skill in literary style and are time-consuming to mark. Further, uniformity of marking of essays is difficult to achieve and it is not possible to test a wide range of knowledge.

Multiple-choice question examinations (MCQs) overcome most of these problems. A wide range of knowledge can be tested and the answers can be computer-marked, thus removing human bias and speeding up the availability of results. The answers can be assessed statistically allowing 'poor questions' – those that are either too easy or too difficult – to be removed from the question bank while retaining those that have a good discriminatory value. Criterion referencing is being introduced into many examinations and the MCQ is ideal for this function.

Infection is a topic which permeates many examinations, both specialist and general. Drs Ross and Emmanuel are to be congratulated on their book, which should prove extremely valuable to trainee microbiologists, public health physicians and clinicians, especially those with an interest in infectious diseases and genitourinary medicine. It will also be valuable for undergraduate students studying for examinations in microbiology/ infection. I can commend this book without reservation to all of these groups.

A. M. Geddes, CBE, MBChB, FRCP, FRCPE, FRCPath, FFPHM

Preface to the Third Edition

Multiple-choice questions are an increasingly important component of examinations in medicine, and most undergraduate examinations and postgraduate fellowship and membership diploma papers contain these in both the UK and elsewhere. Infection and its complications are important in many areas of medical practice and questions on infectious disease and microbiology feature in MCQ papers for membership or fellowship examinations in nearly all fields of medicine. This book is intended to provide sufficient practice in answering such questions.

Of the questions and answers that were included in the first and second editions of this book, over 40% have been updated, amended or replaced in this third edition. Extended answers have been supplied where appropriate to help expand the knowledge of the candidate. They should be looked on as part of the learning process and not treated simply as a checklist.

Medical microbiology and infectious diseases cover a wide range of subjects and we have aimed to be both realistic and practical in the choice of questions using the true/false format. It was not an easy task to compile these and to ensure that the broad field is covered satisfactorily and that the answers provided will satisfy and be agreed by both the active practitioner and the desk-bound purist.

We have not grouped the questions into related areas or topics, e.g. body systems, whether virological or bacteriological, or whether laboratory-based as opposed to clinically-related, because usually no such groupings exist in the real-life examination system. However, to make the exercise rather more manageable and palatable, the 240 questions and answers have been divided into four sections of 60, with a mix of questions in each. The answers and explanations are only a guide and we hope these will stimulate further relevant reading.

Edinburgh, September, 2000

P.W.R.
F.X.S.E.

Section I – Questions

1. *Neisseria meningitidis*:

A. Is the commonest cause of meningitis in infants
B. Antigen may be rapidly detected in the CSF in meningitis
C. Blood cultures are frequently positive in meningitis
D. Vaccines are available for the common serogroups in the UK
E. Treatment of choice is chloramphenicol

2. **Methicillin-resistant *Staphylococcus aureus* (MRSA):**

A. Is usually sensitive to vancomycin
B. Is more likely to cause deep-seated infection
C. Is often resistant to many anti-staphylococcal antibiotics
D. May cause asymptomatic colonisation
E. Usually belongs to phage-type 81

3. **Aminoglycoside antibiotics such as gentamicin:**

A. Act on the bacterial cell wall
B. Are active against staphylococci
C. Are effective in the treatment of severe pneumococcal pneumonia
D. Are contra-indicated in patients with renal impairment
E. May cause loss of visual acuity in the elderly

4. **Airborne spread is important in the transmission of:**

A. Meningococcal meningitis
B. Hepatitis E infection
C. Poliomyelitis
D. Aspergillosis
E. Tuberculosis

5.   In malaria due to *Plasmodium vivax*:

A. Relapsing infection may occur after several months
B. Cerebral malaria is a well-known complication
C. Infection is usually acquired in the Indian sub-continent
D. Diagnosis is usually made by culture of the organism
E. Resistance to antimalarials is common

6.   Causative agents in oral thrush are:

A. *Actinomyces israelii*
B. *Actinomyces naeslundii*
C. *Candida albicans*
D. *Streptococcus mutans*
E. *Bacteroides gingivalis*

7.   In bacterial endocarditis:

A. Blood cultures may be negative
B. Staphylococci are rare causative organisms
C. In the UK incidence is higher in the elderly
D. Combination therapy with a penicillin and an aminoglycoside is advised in most cases
E. Measurement of C-reactive protein in the serum is useful in management

8.   The triple vaccine for the prevention of bacterial infections includes protection against:

A. Diphtheria
B. Pneumonia
C. Tetanus
D. Scarlet fever
E. Infection by *Haemophilus influenzae* type B

9.   Legionnaires' disease:

A. Is easily transmitted from person to person
B. Diagnosis is usually confirmed by serological tests
C. Is caused by an organism that cannot be grown on bacteriological culture media
D. Is treated with a combination of penicillin and gentamicin
E. May present as lobar pneumonia

10. **The triple vaccine for the prevention of virus infections includes protection against:**

A. Rabies virus
B. Polio virus
C. Hepatitis virus
D. Mumps virus
E. Rubella virus

11. **Rotavirus infections:**

A. Are rare in adults
B. Are diagnosed by stool culture
C. Do not require specific antibiotic therapy
D. Can be reliably prevented by immunisation
E. Can be easily spread from person to person

12. **Foetal infections contracted *in utero* can be caused by the following:**

A. *Treponema pallidum*
B. *Corynebacterium diphtheriae*
C. HIV
D. Cytomegalovirus
E. *Toxoplasma gondii*

13. **The haemolytic uraemic syndrome:**

A. Is more common in children
B. In the majority of cases is caused by infection with verotoxin-producing *Escherichia coli*
C. Is rarely associated with haemorrhagic colitis.
D. Is caused by an infective agent that may be transmitted with food
E. Is an indication for urgent antibiotic therapy

14. **The following act as inhibitors of bacterial cell-wall synthesis:**

A. Vancomycin
B. Penicillins
C. Sulphonamides
D. Aminoglycosides
E. Cephalosporins

15. The following act as inhibitors of nucleic acid synthesis in bacteria:

A. Polymyxins
B. Quinolones
C. Tetracyclines
D. Fusidic acid
E. Rifampicin

16. Common causes of meningitis in the neonate include:

A. *Haemophilus influenzae*
B. Coliform organisms
C. Group B streptococci
D. *Staphylococcus aureus*
E. *Streptococcus pneumoniae*

17. Which of the following relate(s) to actinomycosis?

A. Cervico-facial disease is the most common presentation
B. Limited epidemics occur in farming communities
C. Infection is endogenous
D. Antibiotics have no place in therapy
E. Colonies released in pus are called 'sulphur granules'

18. The following have oncogenic properties in humans:

A. Hepatitis B virus
B. Papova viruses
C. Enteroviruses
D. Rabies virus
E. Rubella virus

19. Genital infection with *Candida albicans*:

A. Is more common in pregnancy
B. Can be transmitted sexually
C. Primarily affects the cervix in females
D. Is confirmed by culture on special media
E. Tends to cause persistent infection in immunoglobulin deficiencies

20. In salmonella food poisoning:

A. Symptoms start within 3 hours
B. Antibiotic treatment is not indicated
C. Infected food-handlers are the main source of contamination
D. Diagnosis is usually confirmed by culture of the suspected food.
E. Blood cultures are frequently positive

21. The following bacteria are frequently associated with an acute exacerbation of chronic bronchitis:

A. *Haemophilus influenzae*
B. *Streptococcus mutans*
C. *Streptococcus pneumoniae*
D. *Staphylococcus aureus*
E. *Moraxella (Branhamella) catarrhalis*

22. Laboratory tests helpful in the diagnosis of infectious mono-nucleosis are:

A. The VDRL test
B. The cold agglutinin test
C. The antistreptolysin O titre
D. The heterophile sheep cell antibody test
E. The antinuclear factor (antibody) test

23. Analysis of cerebrospinal fluid from a case of suspected meningitis showed a great increase in protein and a glucose concentration which was 40% of the plasma concentration. The following organisms are unlikely to be the cause:

A. ECHO virus
B. *Mycobacterium tuberculosis*
C. *Streptococcus pneumoniae*
D. *Haemophilus influenzae*
E. *Leptospira icterohaemorrhagiae*

24. Phage typing is a useful procedure in the investigation of outbreaks of infection caused by:

A. *Staphylococcus aureus*
B. *Salmonella typhi*
C. *Mycobacterium tuberculosis*
D. *Salmonella paratyphi* B
E. *Campylobacter* spp

25. The following are recognised causes of gas gangrene in humans:

A. *Clostridium oedematiens*
B. *Clostridium sporogenes*
C. *Clostridium septicum*
D. *Clostridium histolyticum*
E. *Clostridium perfringens*

26. The antistreptolysin O titre is raised in infections caused by:

A. *Enterococcus faecalis*
B. *Streptococcus pneumoniae*
C. *Streptococcus pyogenes*
D. *Streptococcus bovis*
E. *Streptococcus mutans*

27. Organic materials interfere markedly with the bactericidal action of:

A. Ethylene oxide
B. Glutaraldehyde
C. Hypochlorites
D. Gamma irradiation
E. Formalin vapour

28. Lyme disease:

A. Is spread by rat fleas
B. Is a multi-system disorder
C. Is caused by *Borrelia burgdorferi*, a spirochaete
D. Is diagnosed mainly on the basis of serological tests
E. is confined to the northern hemisphere

29. **In a suspected case of poliomyelitis, the most important specimens to be taken for the isolation of the virus are:**

A. Faeces
B. Throat swab
C. Blood
D. Cerebrospinal fluid
E. Urine

30. **The following antimicrobial drugs are effective against penicillinase-producing staphylococci:**

A. Ampicillin or amoxycillin
B. Phenoxymethyl penicillin
C. Imipenem
D. Augmentin (co-amoxiclav)
E. Cefuroxime

31. **Reiter's syndrome is:**

A. Comprised of arthritis, conjunctivitis and urethritis
B. Associated with patchy pneumonia
C. Confirmed by the VDRL test
D. More common in persons who are HLA B8 positive
E. Associated with *Salmonella* infection

32. **Yaws:**

A. Is a sexually-transmitted disease
B. Is treated effectively with penicillin
C. May be transmitted from the mother to the foetus
D. Produces changes in the CSF
E. Diagnosis is confirmed by treponemal (syphilis) serology

33. **Blood cultures are often positive in cases of:**

A. Meningococcal meningitis
B. Bacillary dysentery
C. Primary syphilis
D. Typhoid fever
E. Rheumatic fever

34. Organisms that are important in causing culture-positive infective endocarditis include:

A. *Streptococcus sanguis*
B. *Staphylococcus aureus*
C. *Bacteroides fragilis*
D. *Klebsiella pneumoniae*
E. *Staphylococcus epidermidis*

35. Hyaluronidase production is important in the pathogenicity of:

A. *Clostridium perfringens*
B. *Streptococcus pyogenes*
C. *Streptococcus pneumoniae*
D. *Neisseria gonorrhoeae*
E. *Shigella sonnei*

36. The following spirochaetes produce disease in man:

A. *Borrelia recurrentis*
B. *Borrelia vincenti*
C. *Treponema pertenue*
D. *Leptospira canicola*
E. *Borrelia burgdorferi*

37. The following vaccines contain living organisms

A. BCG
B. Oral polio
C. Hepatitis B
D. Diphtheria
E. Yellow fever

38. Atypical lymphocytosis (mononucleosis) may be a feature of:

A. Epstein–Barr virus infection
B. Influenza B infection
C. Rubella
D. Toxoplasmosis
E. Cytomegalovirus infection

39. Gamma globulins are useful in the prevention of the following infections:

A. Rheumatic fever
B. Gas gangrene
C. Tetanus
D. Rabies
E. Tuberculosis

40. Acute rheumatic fever is:

A. A complication of infection of the throat by *Streptococcus pyogenes*
B. An indication for long-term penicillin prophylaxis
C. Rare in developed countries
D. Prevented by vaccination in childhood
E. Characterised by infective arthritis

41. *Coxiella burneti*:

A. Is a cause of culture-negative infective endocarditis
B. Infection is reliably diagnosed by serological tests
C. Is the cause of Q fever
D. Causes lymphogranuloma venereum
E. Transmission is by insect vectors

42. Trachoma:

A. Is caused by *Mycoplasma* spp
B. Is caused by *Chlamydia*
C. Is common in wet, humid climates
D. Infection often involves the retina
E. Is treated with penicillin

43. Activation of complement can be induced by:

A. IgD
B. IgE
C. IgG
D. IgM
E. IgA

44. T-cell function can be assessed by:

A. Complement fixation tests
B. Polyacrylamide gel electrophoresis
C. Skin-testing
D. Agglutination tests
E. Lymphocyte proliferation

45. B-cell function can be assessed by:

A. Lymph node biopsy
B. Antibody response to tetanus toxoid
C. Peripheral blood white cell counts
D. Serum immunoglobulin levels
E. C-reactive protein estimation

46. Tetanus toxoid

A. Need not be considered after superficial wounds
B. Is given in three doses to infants as a component of a triple vaccine
C. Confers passive immunity
D. Should be avoided in immunocompromised patients
E. Booster doses should be given every three years

47. The following may cause latent infections:

A. Cytomegalovirus (CMV)
B. *Bordetella pertussis*
C. Herpes simplex virus
D. *Clostridium tetani*
E. Varicella-zoster virus

48. Epstein–Barr virus is implicated in:

A. Shingles
B. Burkitt's lymphoma
C. Nasopharyngeal carcinoma
D. Infectious mononucleosis
E. The Creutzfeldt–Jakob syndrome

49. Exotoxins:

A. Are released during the death of bacteria
B. Are polypeptide molecules
C. Can be inactivated by heat
D. Are mainly secreted by Gram-positive bacteria
E. Are rendered non-antigenic by treatment with formalin

50. Endotoxins:

A. May be secreted by Gram-positive bacteria
B. Can be rendered non-toxic by heating to 56°C
C. Activate the complement system
D. Are powerful inducers of antitoxic antibodies
E. Are lipopolysaccharide molecules of which lipid A is the principal toxic factor

51. The following organisms possess capsules:

A. *Haemophilus influenzae*
B. *Cryptosporidium* spp
C. *Streptococcus pneumoniae*
D. *Staphylococcus epidermidis*
E. *Klebsiella pneumoniae*

52. The following are classified as 'viridans streptococci':

A. *Enterococcus faecalis*
B. *Streptococcus pneumoniae*
C. *Streptococcus bovis*
D. *Streptococcus mitior*
E. *Streptococcus agalactiae*

53. The diagnosis of pseudomembranous colitis (PMC) is aided by:

A. Colonoscopic biopsy of lesions
B. Positive blood culture for *Clostridium difficile*
C. Raised antibody levels in blood to *Clostridium difficile*
D. Isolation of *Clostridium difficile* from the stool
E. Detection of *Clostridium difficile* toxin in the stool

54. Blood culture is commonly positive in the following infections:

A. Staphylococcal osteomyelitis
B. Salmonella food poisoning
C. Pneumococcal pneumonia
D. Listeriosis
E. Actinomycosis

55. The more common bacteria causing serious lobar pneumonia following infection with influenza viruses are:

A. *Streptococcus pyogenes*
B. *Streptococcus pneumoniae*
C. *Moraxella (Branhamella) catarrhalis*
D. *Staphylococcus aureus*
E. *Haemophilus influenzae*

56. Macrolides such as erythromycin or clarithromycin are first-line antibiotics in the treatment of infections caused by:

A. *Mycoplasma pneumoniae*
B. *Chlamydia psittaci*
C. *Haemophilus influenzae*
D. *Legionella pneumophila*
E. *Streptococcus pyogenes*

57. Keratoconjunctivitis may be due to infection with:

A. *Borrelia vincenti*
B. *Leptospira icterohaemorrhagiae*
C. Myxoviruses
D. Herpes simplex virus
E. Adenoviruses

58. The following infections in the mother can be transmitted transplacentally and cause foetal damage:

A. Toxoplasmosis
B. Listeriosis
C. Measles
D. Gonorrhoea
E. Cytomegalovirus

59. Infectious mononucleosis:

A. Can be successfully treated with ampicillin
B. Presents most commonly in the pre-school child
C. May be treated by interferon
D. Is caused by herpes simplex virus
E. Is associated with heterophile antibodies in the blood

60. A pet shop owner presented to his doctor with general malaise, headache and fever and was found to have a patchy bronchopneumonia. In the light of his occupation, his illness is likely to be:

A. Psittacosis
B. Mycoplasmal atypical pneumonia
C. Q fever
D. *Haemophilus influenzae* pneumonia
E. Legionnaires' disease

Answers to Section I

1.

A – T The commonest cause in infants (i.e. in the first year of life) was *Haemophilus influenzae* type B (HIB). The use of the HIB vaccine in infancy has greatly reduced the incidence of this infection. In the neonatal period (i.e. the first four weeks of life) *Escherichia coli* and *group B streptococci* are the more common causes of meningitis

B – T Polymerase chain reaction (PCR) for specific meningococcal DNA is also available and is more sensitive than the detection of capsular antigen

C – T

D – F Available vaccines are active only against group C meningococci, and not against group B which is almost as common in the UK

E – F Penicillin is the treatment of choice. Resistance among meningococci is very rare in the UK

2.

A – T May be resistant to many other anti-staphylococcal antibiotics but is usually sensitive to vancomycin. Vancomycin resistance is now described in clinical strains from Japan and elsewhere

B – F Is no more likely to cause deep-seated infections than ordinary *Staphylococcus aureus* strains

C – T

D – T Many patients and staff exposed to these may be colonised asymptomatically in the nose, axillae and groins

E – F May belong to one of several phage types. In fact, phage typing is used to distinguish among strains of MRSA

3.

A – F Act on ribosomes, so interfere with protein synthesis

B – T

C – F Have no activity against streptococci, including *Streptococcus pneumoniae*

D – F Can be used with caution and close monitoring of blood levels

E – F Toxicity is to the vestibular and cochlear branches of the eighth nerve

14

4.

A – T This is true of group A meningococcus, which is very uncommon in temperate countries. Group C and group B meningococci are more likely to be transmitted by close personal contact.

B – F Transmitted by the faeco-oral route, especially via sewage contamination of water supplies.

C – F As in B above

D – T The fungal spores are commonly found as air-borne particles

E – T

5.

A – T In malaria due to *Plasmodium vivax*, exoerythrocytic forms can persist in the liver for months or years

B – F This is true only for *Plasmodium falciparum* ✓

C – T The vast majority of cases of imported vivax malaria are from the Indian sub-continent

D – F The organism cannot be cultured on laboratory media. Diagnosis is made by microscopy of stained smears ✓

E – F This is true only of *Plasmodium falciparum*

6.

A – F

B – F

C – T ·

D – F

E – F

7.

A – T Some cases may be due organisms such as *Coxiella*, *Chlamydia* and *Legionella*, which are difficult to culture

B – F Staphylococci are often the cause of endocarditis, especially on prosthetic valves

C – T

D – T

E – T Useful for monitoring success of therapy

8.
A – T
B – F
C – T
D – F
E – F
The triple vaccine against bacterial diseases contains tetanus toxoid, diphtheria toxoid and killed vaccine against whooping cough (*Bordetella pertussis*)

9.
A – F Usually acquired from environmental sources. Person-to-person transmission is virtually unknown
B – T Indirect immunofluorescence test for antibodies is the most useful
C – F Can be grown on special culture media
D – F Erythromycin, combined with rifampicin in severe cases, is the drug of choice
E – T Typical presentation is a patchy bronchopneumonia but lobar pneumonia occurs in about a third of cases

10.
A – F
B – F
C – F
D – T
E – T
The triple vaccine against viral diseases contains live attenuated vaccines against mumps, measles and rubella

11.
A – F Less common than in children, but outbreaks of infection are not rare in adults
B – F This virus cannot be cultured. Diagnosis is by detecting the virus by electron microscopy or by immunological methods
C – T Diarrhoea is usually self-limiting
D – F Several experimental vaccines have been tried but are not available for routine use
E – T

12.
A – T
B – F
C – T
D – T
E – T

13.
A – T
B – T The commonest strain of verotoxin-producing *Escherichia coli* is O157
C – F Is commonly associated with colitis and bloody diarrhoea
D – T But it is often difficult to isolate the organism from the food
E – F Systemic antibiotic treatment has not been shown to be of clinical benefit

14.
A – T
B – T
C – F Interfere with folate metabolism
D – F Interfere with ribosomal function and hence protein synthesis
E – T

15.
A – F They act on the cell membrane
B – T
C – F Inhibit protein synthesis
D – F Inhibits protein synthesis
E – F

16.
A – F Maternal antibody provides protection during the first 2–3 months of life
B – T Usually *Escherichia coli*
C – T
D – F Rare in the neonatal period
E – F As in D

17.

A – T

B – F Almost always a sporadic disease

C – T

D – F Prolonged course of antibiotics necessary in addition to surgical drainage

E – T

18.

A – T Associated with hepatocellular carcinoma

B – T Associated with genital tract malignancies

C – F

D – F

E – F

19.

A – T

B – T

C – F Affects mainly the vulva and vagina

D – T Cultured on special acid-pH media rich in carbohydrates, e.g. Sabouraud's medium

E – F Persistent infection is commonly associated with deficiency of cell-mediated immunity

20.

A – F Usually takes 24–48 hours. The shorter incubation period is associated with exotoxin-producing organisms such as *Staphylococcus aureus* and *Bacillus cereus*

B – T Self-limiting in most cases

C – F Source is often contaminated food such as poultry, eggs, etc

D – F Usually confirmed by culture of the diarrhoeal stool

E – F Not often positive in food poisoning

21.

A – T

B – F

C – T

D – F Causes exacerbation of cystic fibrosis, but rarely of chronic bronchitis

E – T Particularly as a hospital-acquired infection

22.

A – F Used for the diagnosis of syphilis (Venereal Diseases Reference Laboratory test)

B – F Often positive in mycoplasma infections

C – F Used for the diagnosis of group A streptococcal infections

D – T Also known as the Paul–Bunnell test. 'Monospot' is a rapid commercially-available test for heterophile antibodies

E – F

23.

A – T

B – F Often causes marked elevation of protein and reduced glucose, but the cellular exudate is usually predominantly lymphocytic

C – F

D – F

E – T

24.

A – T

B – T

C – F Phage typing is possible but it is rarely used

D – T

E – F Antigenic types are used

25.

A – T

B – F

C – T

D – T

E – T This is the pathogen most commonly implicated

26.

A – F

B – F

C – T

D – F

E – F

27.
A – F
B – T
C – T
D – F
E – F
The presence of organic material will interfere to a varying extent with all disinfection procedures. Articles for disinfection should be thoroughly cleaned first

28.
A – F Spread by ixodid ('hard') ticks of many wild and domestic animals
B – T Involves skin, joints, nervous system and cardiovascular system
C – T
D – T Though useful, serological tests have low sensitivity and are often falsely-positive
E – T Is widespread in North America and Europe and possibly elsewhere in the Northern Hemisphere

29.
A – T
B – T But less useful than faeces
C – F
D – F
E – F

30.
A – F These agents are destroyed by the staphylococcal penicillinase (β-lactamase)
B – F As above
C – T But is expensive and available only intravenously
D – T
E – T

31.
A – T But all three features may not be present in all cases
B – F
C – F Confirmatory tests not available
D – F Strongly associated with HLA B27
E – T Also associated with other infective diarrhoeas

32.
A – F Usually transmitted by non-sexual physical contact in crowded warm climates
B – T
C – F
D – F CNS infection is rare in yaws
E – T Yaws and syphilis are caused by antigenically very similar organisms

33.
A – T
B – F But *Shigella* spp may very rarely invade the blood stream
C – F But bacteraemia is a feature of secondary syphilis
D – T
E – F

34.
A – T
B – T
C – F Anaerobic organisms very rarely cause endocarditis
D – F 'Coliform' organisms such as *Klebsiella* rarely cause endocarditis
E – T Particularly on prosthetic valves

35.
A – T
B – T
C – F
D – F
E – F

36.
A – T Causes louse-borne relapsing fever
B – T Causes Vincent's angina
C – T Causes yaws. Antigenically similar to *Treponema pallidum*, the cause of syphilis
D – T One of the causative agents of Weil's disease (leptospirosis)
E – T Causes Lyme disease

37.
A – T
B – T
C – F   Made only from the surface antigen component of the virus
D – F   Made from modified exotoxin (toxoid)
E – T

38.
A – T   Causes infectious mononucleosis
B – F
C – T
D – T
E – T

39.
A – F
B – F
C – T   Specific immunoglobulin is useful for immediate prophylaxis of patients who are not adequately immunised with toxoid.
D – T   In post-exposure prophylaxis in combination with active vaccination
E – F

40.
A – T
B – T   To prevent reinfection with *Streptococcus pyogenes*
C – T
D – F   No vaccine available
E – F   The arthritis is non-infective

41.
A – T   Rare but significant cause of serious endocarditis
B – T
C – T
D – F   Lymphogranuloma venereum is caused by certain serotypes of *Chlamydia trachomatis*
E – F   Transmission is by airborne spread

42.
A – F
B – T Caused by *Chlamydia trachomatis*
C – F More common in hot dry climates, e.g. north Africa
D – F Infection affects the conjunctiva only
E – F Resistant to penicillin. Treated with tetracycline or chloram-
        phenicol

43.
A – F
B – F Mediates type1 (anaphylactic) hypersensitivity
C – T
D – T
E – T But aggregates of IgA can activate the alternative pathway of
        complement activation

44.
A – F Complement-fixation tests are used for antibody detection
B – F Polyacrylamide gel electrophoresis is used for separating protein
        fragments
C – T Skin-testing may be used for detecting delayed type hyper-
        sensitivity mediated by T-cells, e.g. the Mantoux test for
        tuberculosis
D – F Agglutination tests are used for detecting antibodies
E – T Mitogen-induced *in vitro* lymphocyte proliferation

45.
A – T
B – T
C – F
D – T
E – F C-reactive protein is an acute-phase protein produced in the liver

46.
A – F Tetanus may follow minor wounds in the unimmunised
B – T Combined with whooping cough and diphtheria vaccines
C – F Induces active humoral (circulating antibody mediated) immunity
D – F Not a live vaccine – made from modified tetanus toxin (toxoid)
E – F Booster doses in adults are required only once every 10 years

47.
A – T
B – F
C – T
D – F
E – T

48.
A – F Shingles is caused by varicella-zoster virus
B – T Association with Burkitt's lymphoma is seen in west Africa
C – T Association with nasopharyngeal carcinoma is seen in south China
D – T Primary infection causes infectious mononucleosis
E – F This is a 'prion' disease, due to an aetiological agent which is thought to be a self-replicating protein. Bovine spongiform encephalopathy (BSE), scrapie in sheep and kuru are other diseases thought to be due to similar agents

49.
A – F
B – T
C – T
D – T
E – F Treatment with formalin renders them non-toxic but they retain antigenicity

50.
A – F Endotoxins are a component of Gram-negative cells
B – F Endotoxins are relatively heat-stable
C – T May activate the complement and clotting systems
D – F Are weak inducers of antitoxic antibodies
E – T

51.
A – T But many strains are non-capsulate
B – F This is a coccidian parasite that may cause diarrhoea. *Cryptococcus neoformans* is a capsulate yeast that causes meningitis
C – T There about 84 capsular serotypes of *Streptococcus pneumoniae*
D – F
E – T

52.
A – F
B – T
C – F
D – T
E – F

53.
A – T Histology is pathognomonic
B – F *Clostridium difficile* infection is not bacteraemic
C – F Antibody tests in blood are not of value in diagnosis
D – T But *Clostridium difficile* can also be isolated from the stool in some normal individuals
E – T But *Clostridium difficile* toxin may also be present in the stool in some normal individuals

54.
A – T
B – F But may be bacteraemic in elderly or debilitated patients
C – T
D – T
E – F Metastatic spread of infection may occur, but bacteraemia is rarely detected

55.
A – T
B – T Probably the most common cause of secondary bacterial pneumonia
C – F Rarely a cause of serious lobar pneumonia
D – T
E – F As in C

56.
A – T
B – T
C – F
D – T But tetracycline seldom used. Rifampicin may be added to erythromycin in serious cases
E – F Antibiotic of choice is penicillin

57.
A – **F**
B – **F** But infection of conjunctiva is often seen
C – **F**
D – **T**
E – **T** Adenoviruses may cause outbreaks of contagious conjunctivitis

58.
A – **T**
B – **T**
C – **F**
D – **F** Gonorrhoea may be transmitted perinatally
E – **T**

59.
A – **F** In fact, ampicillin treatment often results in a characteristic rash
B – **F** Presents most commonly in young adults
C – **F** No long-term benefits demonstrated
D – **F** Is caused by the Epstein–Barr virus
E – **T** Heterophile antibodies used in the Paul–Bunnell test

60.
A – **T**
B – **F**
C – **F**
D – **F**
E – **F**

Section II – Questions

61. **Administration of gamma globulin is indicated in the following:**

A. Prophylaxis of tetanus
B. Treatment of Vincent's infection of the throat
C. Prophylaxis of chicken pox
D. Treatment of hepatitis A infection
E. Treatment of hepatitis B infection

62. **Mycoplasmas:**

A. Are resistant to penicillin
B. Are often present as commensals
C. Can be grown on laboratory media
D. Have a cell wall
E. Are susceptible to erythromycin

63. **The following organisms causing infections in man may be acquired as a result of eating inadequately cooked meat:**

A. *Trichomonas* spp
B. *Plasmodium vivax*
C. *Toxoplasma* spp
D. *Taenia saginata*
E. *Trichinella spiralis*

64. **The Arthus reaction in man:**

A. Is an acute inflammatory response
B. May be severe if circulating antibody levels are high
C. May occur after pneumococcal vaccination
D. Occurs within half an hour of exposure
E. Is mediated by IgE

65. The following are examples of immunological tests used for demonstrating antigen–antibody reactions *in vivo*:

A. Haemagglutination inhibition (HAI)
B. Skin test for tuberculosis
C. Enzyme-linked immunosorbent assay (ELISA)
D. Skin test for penicillin hypersensitivity
E. Radioimmunoassay (RIA)

66. Intestinal amoebae:

A. Commonly parasitise the jejunum and ileum
B. Consist mostly of pathogenic species
C. May cause peritonitis
D. Are susceptible to metronidazole
E. May cause liver abscesses

67. Endotoxin can produce:

A. Circulatory collapse
B. Activation of the complement cascade
C. Disseminated intravascular coagulation (DIC)
D. Fever
E. Granulomas

68. Immunisation against hepatitis B infection will also protect against infection by the following viruses:

A. Hepatitis A
B. Hepatitis C
C. Hepatitis D
D. Hepatitis E
E. HTLV I and II

69. Hepatitis C virus :

A. Is responsible for chronic liver disease in 50% of those infected
B. Causes jaundice in a minority of infected persons
C. Is a major cause of transfusion-associated hepatitis
D. Is an aetiological agent in hepatocellular carcinoma
E. Is transmitted by arthropod vectors

70. Hepatitis A virus infection:

A. Has an incubation period of 5–10 days
B. Is transmitted by sexual intercourse
C. Is a common precursor of chronic liver disease
D. Confers long-lasting immunity
E. Can be prevented by the use of killed vaccines

71. A raised titre of anti-HBs in the blood:

A. Signifies previous hepatitis B infection
B. Is produced after hepatitis B vaccination
C. Indicates immunity to hepatitis B infection
D. Occurs during the incubation period of hepatitis B infection
E. Indicates active hepatitis B infection

72. Reliable diagnoses of infections caused by the following viruses may be made in the laboratory within 24 hours of receiving the appropriate specimen:

A. Respiratory syncytial virus
B. Rotavirus
C. Herpes simplex virus
D. Coxsackie virus
E. Cytomegalovirus

73. The herpes group of viruses includes:

A. Varicella-zoster virus
B. Papilloma virus
C. Rabies virus
D. Epstein–Barr virus
E. Cytomegalovirus

74. In toxoplasmosis:

A. Antimicrobial therapy may not be required
B. The cat is a primary animal host of *Toxoplasma gondii*
C. Infection is contracted via the respiratory route
D. Most infections in man are asymptomatic
E. Serology is the most useful method of diagnosis

75. Zoonoses transmitted by unpasteurised milk include:

A. Brucellosis
B. Leptospirosis
C. Q fever
D. Listeriosis
E. Verotoxin-producing *Escherichia coli* such as *E. coli* O157

76. Zoonoses of viral aetiology include:

A. Lassa fever
B. Q fever
C. Chlamydial infection
D. Orf
E. Hantavirus infection

77. Useful drugs in fungal infections are:

A. Ribavirin
B. Amantidine
C. Terbinafine
D. Fluconazole
E. Itraconazole

78. Viruses associated with the production of vesicular lesions include:

A. Respiratory syncytial
B. Herpes simplex
C. Coxsackie
D. Papova
E. Hepatitis A

79. Candida albicans:

A. Infection is effectively treated with broad-spectrum antibiotics
B. Can be seen on Gram's stain
C. Requires anaerobic conditions for growth in the laboratory
D. Causes granuloma inguinale
E. Is a cause of oesophagitis

80. Gram-negative bacilli include:

A. *Salmonella*
B. *Klebsiella*
C. *Listeria*
D. *Corynebacterium*
E. *Campylobacter*

81. Gram-positive bacterial genera include:

A. *Brucella*
B. *Lactobacillus*
C. *Bacteroides*
D. *Neisseria*
E. *Yersinia*

82. Genital herpes infection:

A. May be caused by herpes simplex virus type 1
B. Usually results in long-lasting immunity
C. Is always symptomatic
D. Can be treated effectively with a ten-day course of acyclovir
E. May produce spontaneous abortion

83. Bacteria associated with food poisoning are:

A. *Helicobacter pylori*
B. *Clostridium perfringens*
C. *Streptococcus pyogenes*
D. *Pseudomonas aeruginosa*
E. *Bacillus cereus*

84. The polymerase chain reaction (PCR)

A. Is a rapid test for the detection of specific bacterial proteins in tissues and body fluids
B. Is useful for obtaining rapid antimicrobial susceptibility results
C. May be used to detect specific RNA as well as DNA
D. May be used for tests on stored tissue samples
E. Is not suitable for routine diagnostic use

85. Skin tests are of diagnostic significance in:

A. Diphtheria
B. Syphilis
C. Tuberculosis
D. Typhoid fever
E. Hydatid disease

86. Production of exotoxin is an important factor in the patho-genicity of:

A. *Escherichia coli*
B. *Clostridium botulinum*
C. *Mycobacterium tuberculosis*
D. *Corynebacterium diphtheriae*
E. *Vibrio cholerae*

87. Fungi associated with superficial skin infections include:

A. *Aspergillus* spp
B. *Histoplasma capsulatum*
C. *Microsporum* spp
D. *Cryptococcus neoformans*
E. *Trichophyton* spp

88. The following are examples of DNA viruses:

A. Herpes simplex virus
B. Papilloma virus
C. Influenza viruses
D. Enteroviruses
E. Epstein–Barr virus

89. Water-borne infections include:

A. Poliomyelitis
B. Schistosomiasis
C. Cryptosporidiosis
D. Leptospirosis
E. Actinomycosis

90. Pseudomembranous colitis:

A. Is caused by *Clostridium novyi*
B. Is mediated by an exotoxin
C. Is common in children
D. Can result from hospital cross-infection
E. Cannot be treated with antibiotics

91. Uveitis is a feature of:

A. Toxoplasmosis
B. Reiter's disease
C. Hepatitis B infection
D. Diphtheria
E. Tuberculosis

92. C-reactive protein (CRP):

A. Does not have antigen specificity
B. Levels increase significantly in acute viral infections
C. Is produced in the liver
D. Measurement is useful in the management of bacterial endocarditis
E. Activates complement by the classical pathway

93. Pneumococcal vaccine:

A. Should be administered on an annual basis
B. Is made from cell-wall antigen from several serotypes
C. Is given intradermally
D. Is particularly important for persons who have had splenectomy
E. Is ineffective in the elderly

94. The following virus infections are transmitted by the faeco-oral route:

A. Hepatitis A
B. Hepatitis B
C. Hepatitis C
D. Hepatitis D
E. Hepatitis E

95. Coagulase-negative staphylococci:

A. Produce extracellular slime which may contribute to pathogenicity
B. Are commensals on the skin
C. Are an important cause of infection associated with indwelling prosthetic devices
D. Produce an enzyme which coagulates plasma
E. Include *Staphylococcus saprophyticus*, a common cause of urinary tract infection

96. *Pseudomonas aeruginosa:*

A. Frequently causes lung infection in patients with cystic fibrosis.
B. Is naturally resistant to many antibiotics
C. Produces exotoxins which contribute to virulence
D. Frequently causes septicaemia in patients with AIDS
E. Is not sensitive to β-lactam antibiotics

97. In whooping cough:

A. Flucloxacillin is effective in treatment
B. Infection is spread by asymptomatic carriers
C. Diagnosis is confirmed by isolating the organism from throat swabs during the acute stage of illness
D. A full course of vaccination gives long-lasting immunity
E. Infection before the age of 3 months is rare because of protection afforded by maternal antibodies

98. *Enterococcus faecalis:*

A. Is a cause of infective endocarditis
B. Is included in the common term 'viridans streptococci'
C. Possesses Lancefield group D carbohydrate antigen
D. Is highly susceptible to penicillin
E. Is associated with a form of food poisoning

99. The following are true of immunisation:

A. A full course of hepatitis B vaccination gives protection for only 1–2 years
B. Oral polio vaccine is not advised for patients with AIDS
C. Anti-tetanus immunoglobulin and tetanus toxoid can be given at the same time for prevention of tetanus
D. National eradication of rubella can be effectively achieved by giving the vaccine to girls at secondary school entry
E. The oral typhoid vaccine is as effective as the parenteral vaccine

100. Bacteria responsible for community-acquired pneumonia include:

A. *Streptococcus pneumoniae*
B. *Legionella pneumophila*
C. *Pseudomonas aeruginosa*
D. *Mycoplasma pneumoniae*
E. *Chlamydia trachomatis*

101. In diphtheria:

A. The pathogenesis is mediated by exotoxin
B. The primary site of infection is always the throat
C. Immunisation is very effective in prevention
D. Blood culture is usually positive
E. The causative organism has been eradicated in the UK

102. In pregnancy:

A. Immunisation of the mother against tetanus should be avoided
B. If tuberculosis is diagnosed in the mother, treatment should be delayed until after the birth
C. Infection of the mother with hepatitis A virus causes congenital abnormalities
D. Tetracycline therapy should be avoided
E. The mother can be safely immunised with oral (Sabin) polio vaccine

103. Poliomyelitis:

A. Is caused by an enterovirus
B. Is diagnosed by a four-fold rise in neutralising antibody
C. May be spread by both faeco–oral and respiratory routes
D. May be associated with aseptic meningitis
E. Killed vaccine is no longer of any value in prevention

104. The following are examples of 'prion' diseases:

A. Infectious polyneuritis (Guillain–Barré syndrome)
B. Creutzfeldt–Jakob syndrome
C. Bovine spongiform encephalitis
D. Kuru
E. Subacute sclerosing panencephalitis (SSPE)

105. The following are causes of food- or water-borne infection:

A. *Bacillus cereus*
B. *Yersinia enterocolitica*
C. *Giardia lamblia*
D. *Clostridium difficile*
E. *Listeria monocytogenes*

106. Viruses that can cause sexually-transmitted diseases include:

A. ECHO
B. Herpes simplex
C. Papilloma virus
D. Hepatitis A
E. Hepatitis B

107. Features of childhood meningococcal meningitis include:

A. Raised glucose level in the CSF
B. Presence of Gram-negative diplococci in CSF smears
C. Raised polymorphonuclear cell count in the CSF
D. Septicaemia
E. A good response to treatment with aminoglycoside antibiotics

108. Infective endocarditis:

A. Affects only damaged heart valves
B. Is rarely caused by enterococci
C. Can usually be confirmed by blood culture
D. May be caused by viruses
E. Often occurs on prosthetic valves

109. Myocarditis may be caused by:

A. *Staphylococcus aureus*
B. Enteroviruses
C. *Corynebacterium diphtheriae*
D. *Streptococcus pyogenes*
E. *Toxoplasma gondii*

110. Complications of measles include:

A. Subacute sclerosing panencephalitis (SSPE)
B. Bacterial pneumonia
C. Epididymo-orchitis
D. Haemorrhagic skin rashes
E. Congenital abnormalities

111. Acute osteomyelitis:

A. Is usually caused by haematogenous spread
B. Is most commonly caused by *Staphylococcus aureus*
C. Is often associated with *Haemophilus influenzae* in children
D. Frequently affects more than one bone
E. Often yields positive blood cultures

112. Antibiotics contraindicated in pregnancy include:

A. Aminoglycosides
B. Cefuroxime
C. Tetracyclines
D. Clarithromycin
E. Phenoxymethyl penicillin

113. In influenza:

A. The causative viruses can be grown in tissue culture
B. The vaccines include all the current antigenic types
C. A rapid diagnosis can be made by direct immuno-fluorescent tests
D. Treatment with amantidine is effective
E. Pneumococcal pneumonia is a common complication

114. In salmonella food poisoning:

A. Diagnosis is usually made by culturing faeces from infected persons
B. *Salmonella enteritidis* is a common aetiological agent
C. Antibiotic treatment is not usually indicated
D. Poultry is the commonest source of infection
E. Symptoms begin within 2–3 hours of eating contaminated food

115. Bovine spongiform encephalopathy:

A. Is caused by an agent that is killed by pasteurisation
B. Can be prevented by vaccination of cattle
C. Has been shown to be transmissible to humans
D. Was transmitted to cattle by contaminated feed
E. Is caused by an agent related to RNA viruses

116. In *Campylobacter* infection:

A. Person-to-person spread is common in outbreaks
B. Poultry is a common source
C. Antibiotic treatment is usually not indicated
D. The most common cause of community-acquired diarrhoea
E. Watery diarrhoea is a common presentation

117. Lyme disease:

A. Principally affects the skin and joints
B. May result from infection with many species of the genus *Borrelia*
C. Is transmitted by fleas living on wild mammals
D. Diagnosis is by blood culture using special media
E. Is not improved by antibiotic therapy

118. Rabies:

A. Produces a fatal spongiform encephalopathy
B. The main reservoir of infection in Europe is unvaccinated dogs
C. May spread from person to person by close contact
D. Is prevented by the use of a live vaccine
E. Has been eradicated in the UK

119. Leptospirosis:

A. May be acquired from cattle
B. Is often diagnosed by positive blood cultures
C. Is not preventable by vaccination in man
D. Diagnosis is confirmed by detecting serum antibodies
E. Is usually a self-limiting disease

120. *Pneumocystis carinii*:

A. Is classified as a fungus
B. May be present asymptomatically in healthy adults
C. Infection is diagnosed by serological tests
D. Produces disease only in patients with specific T-cell loss
E. May be isolated by blood culture using special mycological culture media

Answers to Section II

61.
A – T For contaminated wounds in patients not up-to-date with their tetanus immunisation.
B – F
C – T For post-exposure prophylaxis in non-immune patients at special risk from infection, e.g. in pregnancy
D – F May be used in prophylaxis
E – F As in D

62.
A – T Infections are usually treated with erythromycin or tetracyclines
B – T
C – T
D – F
E – T

63.
A – F These organisms cause genito-urinary infections, e.g. *Trichomonas vaginalis*
B – F
C – T Cat is the primary reservoir, but transmission to humans often occurs through consumption of infected lamb or pork
D – T This is the beef tapeworm
E – T Causes trichinellosis, transmitted through pork

64.
A – T
B – T
C – T particularly true with revaccination, if high titres to some of the serotypes persist from the previous vaccination
D – F Several hours or days
E – F IgG or IgM

The Arthus reaction is a localised antigen–antibody reaction at the site of introduction of antigen in individuals with high circulating levels of the corresponding antibody, e.g. local reaction to tetanus toxoid in individuals who are already immune; farmer's lung

65.

A – F
B – F Tuberculin skin tests measure cell mediated hypersensitivity
C – F
D – T Detects circulating penicillin-specific IgE
E – F

All these tests except B and D are *in vitro* tests for quantifying antibodies

66.

A – F Pathogenic amoebae mainly affect the colon (*Entamoeba histolytica*)
B – F Most species are non-pathogenic, e.g. *Entamoeba coli, Entamoeba nana*
C – T Usually as a result of ruptured amoebic liver abscess
D – T
E – T

67.

A – T
B – T
C – T
D – T
E – F

68.

A – F
B – F
C – T The hepatitis D agent (delta agent) can replicate only in the presence of the hepatitis B virus
D – F
E – F

69.

A – T
B – T
C – T
D – F Hepatocellular carcinoma is associated with hepatitis B
E – F Transmitted parenterally or by sexual contact

70.
A – F Incubation period ranges from 15 to 45 days
B – F Transmission is faeco–oral
C – F Recovery is usually complete
D – T
E – T Formalin-killed vaccine available

71.
A – T
B – T
C – T
D – F
E – F

72.
A – T By direct immunofluorescence
B – T By electron microscopy or SDS-PAGE
C – T By direct immunofluorescence
D – F Cell culture or animal inoculation is required
E – T By the presence of characteristic inclusion bodies

73.
A – T
B – F This belongs to the papovaviridae
C – F This belongs to the rhabdoviridae
D – T
E – T

74.
A – T Most cases recover without specific antimicrobial treatment, but treatment with pyrimethamine is required if there is retinitis or myocarditis
B – T Cats are the primary source of oocysts but many domestic and wild animals can be sources of tissue cysts infective to man
C – F Transmission is by ingestion of tissue cysts or oocysts
D – T
E – T

75.
A – T
B – F Inoculation through abraded skin or mucous membranes
C – T
D – T
E – T

76.
A – T Rodent reservoir
B – F Caused by *Coxiella burneti* – not a virus
C – F
D – T Caused by accidental inoculation of a sheep poxvirus
E – T Rodent reservoir

77.
A – F Antiviral agent sometimes useful in treating respiratory syncytial virus infection
B – F Antiviral agent useful in treating influenza A infection
C – T Useful for treating fungal nail infections
D – T Oral or parenterally available agent particularly useful for treatment of infections with yeasts such as *Candida albicans* or *Cryptococcus* spp
E – T Broad-spectrum antifungal agent

78.
A – F
B – T
C – T Cause vesicular pharyngeal lesions called herpangina
D – F Cause wart-like lesions
E – F

79.
A – F These often predispose to *Candida* infection
B – T
C – F
D – F
E – T

80.
A – T
B – T
C – F Gram-positive bacilli
D – F As above
E – T Gram-negative curved bacilli

81.
A – F
B – T
C – F
D – F These are Gram-negative cocci
E – F

82.
A – T Though more commonly due to type 2
B – F Recurrent infections are not uncommon
C – F Is often asymptomatic
D – T But treatment must be started early
E – F

83.
A – F
B – T Associated with meat-based foods
C – T But very uncommon
D – F
E – T Associated with cooked rice

84.
A – F Detects specific DNA or RNA sequences, not proteins
B – F Antimicrobial susceptibility tests require growth of viable whole organisms. However, certain mutant DNA sequences which confer specific antibiotic resistance may be detected by PCR (e.g. rifampicin resistance in *Mycobacterium tuberculosis*)
C – T
D – T However, RNA is far less stable than DNA and stored tissues are not suitable for PCR tests based on RNA amplification
E – F Is now used increasingly in diagnostic microbiology

85.

A – F　The Schick test may be used for detecting immunity, but is not of diagnostic value in suspected cases

B – F　Diagnosis is made by serology

C – T　Mantoux, Heaf or Tine tests

D – F　Diagnosis is based on blood culture or stool culture

E – T　But this test is of low sensitivity and specificity and is no longer used. More sensitive and specific serological tests are now available

86.

A – T　In verotoxin-producing strains, e.g. *Escherichia coli* O157

B – T　Disease is due to exotoxin released by the bacterium in the contaminated food

C – F

D – T　Diphtheria toxin causes local tissue necrosis as well as systemic toxicity including myocardiotoxicity

E – T

87.

A – F　Usually associated with lung infections and disseminated infections in immunocompromised patients

B – F　As in A

C – T

D – F　Usually associated with meningitis and disseminated infections in immunocompromised patients

E – T

88.

A – T

B – T

C – F

D – F

E – T

89.

A – T　By ingestion of faecally-contaminated water

B – T　By swimming in water infested with infected snails

C – T　As in A, but the source of contamination is often cattle

D – T　By contact with water fouled by infected animals

E – F

90.

A – F Caused by *Clostridium difficile*

B – T Mucosal damage is caused by a cytotoxin secreted by the organism

C – F The disease is very rare in children even though the organism may be often present in the gut

D – T

E – F Vancomycin or metronidazole is given orally in severe cases

91.

A – T

B – T

C – F

D – F

E – T

92.

A – T

B – F Viral infections do not usually elicit a CRP response; bacterial infections often do

C – T Secreted by hepatocytes

D – T It is a useful objective parameter for monitoring progress

E – F Does not involve the complement system

93.

A – F Once every 5 years is adequate

B – F Made from capsular polysaccharide antigen of several serotypes

C – F Given intramuscularly

D – T

E – F Often effective in the elderly

94.

A – T

B – F

C – F

D – F

E – T

95.
A – T Enables the organism to adhere to the site of infection
B – T
C – T Are by far the most important pathogens infecting prosthetic heart valves, joint replacements, indwelling vascular catheters, etc
D – F Coagulase production is a property of coagulase-positive staphylococci (*Staphylococcus aureus*)
E – T

96.
A – T The mucoid forms are particularly difficult to treat. Other pathogens involved in cystic fibrosis include *Staphylococcus aureus*, *Haemophilus influenzae* and *Pseudomonas cepacia*
B – T
C – T
D – F *Pseudomonas* septicaemias are more likely to occur in granulocytopaenic patients
E – F Third-generation cephalosporins and other β-lactam antibiotics such as piperacillin, azlocillin, etc are active against most strains of *Pseudomonas aeruginosa*

97.
A – F Erythromycin is the preferred antibiotic
B – F There is no asymptomatic carrier state in pertussis
C – F Pernasal swabs are preferred
D – F Immunity declines rapidly over the course of a few years
E – F Infection in early infancy is not uncommon

98.
A – T Particularly in the elderly
B – F These do not produce partial (green) haemolysis
C – T
D – F Is generally much less susceptible than other streptococci
E – F

99.

A – F Protective levels of antibody persist for at least 5 years after successful immunisation.

B – T Live vaccines in general should be avoided in all patients with severe T-cell deficiency

C – T

D – F Universal immunisation including boys is necessary to achieve eradication. This is current policy in the UK using the MMR (mumps, measles and rubella) vaccine

E – T

100.

A – T The commonest cause

B – T An uncommon but important cause

C – F

D – T Another common cause

E – F *Chlamydia trachomatis* is a rare cause of hospital acquired pneumonia in neonates. However, *Chlamydia pneumoniae*, a newly recognised organism, is increasingly recognised as a cause of community-acquired pneumonia

101.

A – T The tissue necrosis at the site of infection and the cardiotoxic effects are mediated by the diphtheria toxin

B – F Infection may occasionally present as necrotic ulcers at other sites

C – T

D – F There is no invasion of deep tissue by the pathogen, *Corynebacterium diphtheriae*. Clinical disease is due to the effects of the exotoxin

E – F Though rare, toxigenic strains of *Corynebacterium diphtheriae* are still occasionally isolated in the UK. Clinical cases of diphtheria, however, have only been due to imported infections in recent years, particularly from countries of the former Soviet Union

102.

A – F This is not a live vaccine

B – F The risks of delaying the treatment are much higher than the teratogenic risks of the chemotherapy

C – F

D – T Dental discolouration in baby; maternal hepatotoxicity.

E – F All live vaccines should be avoided in pregnancy

103.
A – T

B – T But the mainstay of laboratory diagnosis is virus isolation from throat swab or stool sample

C – T But the faeco–oral route is by far the most important

D – T

E – F It is used in situations where live vaccines are contraindicated, e.g. pregnancy or in the immunocompromised

104.
A – F

B – T

C – T This agent is thought to cause new-variant CJD in humans

D – T

E – F This is a complication of measles

'Prion' diseases are thought to be due to a self-replicating protein agent(s) which lacks DNA or RNA. Pathologically they present as slowly-developing but fatal spongiform encephalopathy

105.
A – T Causes outbreaks of food poisoning especially associated with rice-based foods

B – T Milk, meat and drinking water have been implicated

C – T Cysts of the organism are resistant to water chlorination

D – F

E – T Pâtés, soft-cheeses and other dairy products particularly if prepared from unpasteurised raw materials and stored with inadequate refrigeration

106.
A – F

B – T Genital herpes

C – T Genital warts

D – F

E – T

107.

A – F CSF glucose levels are reduced to 60% or less compared to plasma levels taken at the same time

B – T

C – T

D – T Often with a purpuric or haemorrhagic rash in which meningococci may be detected

E – F Treatment of choice is penicillin

108.

A – F Apparently normal valves may also be affected, particularly by virulent organisms like *Staphylococcus aureus*

B – F Enterococci are a frequent cause, particularly in the elderly

C – T Positive in more than 95% of untreated cases

D – F Difficult-to-grow organisms like *Coxiella*, *Chlamydia* or *Legionella* may occasionally be responsible but true viruses are not implicated

E – T Endocarditis is a well-known complication of valve replacement when it is most frequently due to coagulase-negative staphylococci

109.

A – T Often as a complication of endocarditis, in the form of myocardial abscess

B – T Coxsackie, ECHO and polio are enteroviruses which can cause myocarditis

C – T The exotoxin causes a toxic myocarditis

D – T Rheumatic fever and myocarditis are a complication of streptococcal pharyngitis

E – T Myocarditis is an uncommon but serious complication of toxoplasmosis

110.

A – T

B – T Particularly in malnourished children

C – F This is a complication of mumps

D – T Rash is usually maculo–papular, but haemorrhagic skin rashes may rarely occur as a hypersensitivity phenomenon during reinfection in the partially immune

E – F

111.

A – T

B – T

C – F *Haemophilus influenzae* type B was an important cause in children aged 0–4 years before the introduction of vaccination. It is still common in countries where vaccination against *H. influenzae* type B (HIB) is not provided

D – F Frequently affects only one bone, but dissemination due to septi-caemia to other sites including bone may occur if treatment is delayed

E – T Blood culture is nearly always positive

112.

A – T 8th nerve and renal toxicity

B – F

C – T Dental staining and maternal hepatotoxicity

D – F

E – F

113.

A – T

B – T Vaccine used is developed specifically each year for currently prevalent antigenic types

C – T Nasopharyngeal aspirates, nose swabs, throat swabs or sputum may be used

D – F Only useful for prophylaxis (influenza A only)

E – T Other serious bacterial pneumonias such as *Staphylococcus aureus* or group A streptococcal pneumonia may also occur as complications

114.

A – T The food sample is seldom available for examination

B – T

C – T Usually a self-limiting infection. Antibiotic treatment may be indicated in bacteraemic cases or in the elderly and immuno-compromised. Antibiotics may also be used in hospital outbreaks to limit person-to-person spread

D – T Poultry meat, eggs and egg-based foods

E – F Symptoms usually begin 24–48 hours after eating contaminated food

115.

A – F The causative agent may survive autoclaving

B – F No vaccine is available

C – T Though this has not been formally proven in humans, there is now strong evidence for this. Nerve tissue and offal are now prohibited from use in human or animal food production

D – T But this is no longer the case, after the introduction of the ban on the use of animal offal in the production of animal feed

E – F The agent is not related to any known virus and does not contain DNA or RNA. It is thought to be a self-replicating protein

116.

A – F Person-to-person spread is rare but may occur, for example, in mothers looking after infected children with diarrhoea

B – T The vast majority of poultry flocks in the UK are infected

C – T But erythromycin may be useful in cases with severe symptoms

D – T Commonest causative organism in cases where a bacteriological diagnosis is made

E – T But may vary from a few loose stools to severe bloody diarrhoea

117.

A – F Many organ systems may be affected in addition to these, particularly the nervous system, the musculoskeletal system and the heart

B – F Though there are strain differences, there is only one species so far recognised to be associated with Lyme disease, *Borrelia burgdorferi*

C – F The vectors are ixodid (hard) ticks, not fleas

D – F Blood culture for *Borrelia burgdorferi* is used only as a research method

E – F Antibiotic therapy produces a good response particularly in the early stages of infection (amoxycillin, tetracycline or ceftriaxone for 4 weeks)

118.

A – F Does not produce spongiform changes in brain tissue, but characteristic cytoplasmic inclusion bodies (Negri bodies) are seen

B – F The main reservoir of infection in Europe is in wild canines such as the fox

C – T Person-to-person spread by close contact may occur, but only very rarely

D – F The vaccine in use is inactivated (killed) human diploid cell cultures of vaccine strain

E – T Though not in Europe

119.

A – T Leptospirosis is an occupational hazard among farm-workers
B – F Routine blood culture media do not support the growth of *Leptospira* spp
C – T
D – T
E – T Leptospirosis is a mild illness in most cases

120.

A – T
B – T
C – F Antibodies are frequently found in normal persons
D – F Disease was first described in severely malnourished children
E – F

Section III – Questions

121. Cryptosporidiosis:

A. Is usually a self-limiting disease
B. May be acquired by person-to-person transmission
C. Is usually an infection of immunocompromised patients
D. Is diagnosed by detection of oocysts in the stool sample
E. May occur as water-borne outbreaks

122. Acute gastroenteritis commonly accompanies infection with the following:

A. Caliciviruses
B. ECHO virus
C. Hepatitis A
D. Rotavirus
E. Coxsackie virus

123. The common cold syndrome may be caused by:

A. Cytomegalovirus
B. Adenovirus
C. Parainfluenza virus
D. Rotavirus
E. Respiratory syncytial virus

124. Bacterial pathogens that may be carried asymptomatically in the upper respiratory tract include:

A. *Bordetella pertussis*
B. *Neisseria meningitidis*
C. *Haemophilus influenzae* type B
D. Group A haemolytic streptococci
E. *Mycobacterium tuberculosis*

125. In hepatitis A infection:

A. Virus is excreted in significant amounts only after jaundice appears
B. Chronic carriage occurs in around 30% of cases
C. Spread is mainly by contaminated food and water
D. Prevention is by a live vaccine
E. Diagnosis is usually confirmed by serology

126. Viral hepatitis may be caused by:

A. Coxsackie virus
B. Cytomegalovirus
C. Epstein–Barr virus
D. Herpes simplex virus
E. Polio virus

127. Mumps:

A. Can be prevented by a live vaccine
B. Diagnosis can be confirmed by serology
C. Is caused by a paramyxovirus
D. May be complicated by oophoritis
E. Most commonly affects the submandibular salivary glands

128. In human tuberculosis:

A. *Mycobacterium bovis* may cause pulmonary disease
B. A killed vaccine is used to prevent disease
C. Modern antibiotic treatment usually includes an aminoglycoside agent
D. *Mycobacterium avium-intracellulare* is a common cause in patients with AIDS
E. Immunity is mainly due to humoral antibodies

129. Candidiasis is associated with:

A. Treatment with broad-spectrum antibiotics
B. Diabetes mellitus
C. Hospital cross-infection
D. AIDS
E. Use of intra-uterine contraceptive devices

130. In acute exacerbations of chronic obstructive airways diseases (COAD):

A. Staphylococci are common pathogens
B. *Streptococcus pneumoniae* is rarely a cause
C. Culture of sputum is diagnostic
D. C-reactive protein levels are raised
E. *Haemophilus influenzae* is commonly associated

131. Children with the following conditions should not be given the MMR vaccine:

A. Congenital heart disease
B. A history of anaphylaxis
C. HIV infection
D. Cystic fibrosis
E. Down's syndrome

132. Hepatitis B:

A. Is a DNA virus
B. Produces chronic hepatitis in 5–10% of cases
C. Infection has a shorter incubation than hepatitis A
D. Is sexually transmitted
E. Infection is prevented by the use of a sub-unit vaccine

133. *Staphylococcus aureus* has a well-established association with:

A. Toxic epidermal necrolysis
B. Cholecystitis
C. Toxic shock syndrome
D. Acute osteomyelitis
E. Food poisoning

134. In typhoid fever:

A. More than one species of *Salmonella* may be implicated
B. Less than 10% of treated patients will become chronic carriers
C. The carrier state may be eradicated by prolonged antibiotic therapy
D. Serology is useful in diagnosis
E. Prevention may be achieved by a live oral vaccine

135. *Candida albicans* is a well-established aetiological agent in:

A. Hand, foot and mouth disease
B. Denture stomatitis
C. Oesophagitis
D. Cold sores
E. Vincent's angina

136. Viruses causing vesicular rashes are:

A. Herpes simplex
B. Measles
C. Rubella
D. Varicella-zoster
E. Epstein–Barr

137. Herpes simplex virus is associated with:

A. Encephalitis
B. Keratoconjunctivitis
C. Whitlow
D. Acute stomatitis
E. Primary atypical pneumonia

138. Food poisoning may be caused by the ingestion of foods containing preformed exotoxins produced by:

A. *Bacillus cereus*
B. *Listeria monocytogenes*
C. *Salmonella enteritidis*
D. *Clostridium difficile*
E. *Staphylococcus aureus*

139. Killed whole organisms are used in vaccines for the prevention of:

A. Tuberculosis
B. Whooping cough
C. Typhoid
D. Mumps
E. Tetanus

140. The secretory IgA class of antibody:

A. Is responsible for type 1 hypersensitivity
B. Activates complement by the classical pathway
C. Is found in the saliva and tears
D. Confers immunity on mucosal surfaces
E. Appears as a dimer at the site of action

141. Continuous long-term antimicrobial prophylaxis is indicated

A. For patients with prosthetic heart valves
B. Following acute rheumatic fever
C. In recurrent vulvo-vaginitis with herpes simplex infection
D. Following splenectomy
E. For suppression of recurrent urinary tract infections in patients with long-term urinary catheters

142. *Streptococcus pneumoniae*:

A. Is a common aetiological agent in meningitis
B. Is invariably sensitive to penicillin
C. Infections can be prevented by vaccination
D. On Gram-staining appears as Gram-positive cocci in clumps
E. Has a characteristic polysaccharide capsule

143. Methods used for detecting antibodies include:

A. Indirect immunofluorescence
B. Coagulase test
C. Haemagglutination inhibition
D. Enzyme-linked immunoassay (EIA)
E. Polymerase chain reaction

144. Metronidazole is

A. Absorbed well when given orally
B. Safe in pregnancy
C. Effective against many protozoan parasites
D. Indicated for the treatment of pseudomembranous colitis
E. Not easily transported across the blood-brain barrier

145. The following pathogens cause zoonoses involving cattle:

A. *Leptospira* spp
B. *Cryptosporidium* spp
C. *Mycobacterium tuberculosis*
D. *Escherichia coli* O-157
E. *Brucella abortus*

146. Clostridium difficile:

A. May occasionally be found as part of the commensal flora of the gut
B. Produces two separate exotoxins
C. Toxins, when detected in the stool sample, are pathognomonic of pseudomembranous colitis
D. Is an obligate anaerobe
E. Causes outbreaks of nosocomial (hospital-acquired) diarrhoea

147. Enveloped DNA viruses include:

A. Varicella-zoster
B. Rhinovirus
C. Cytomegalovirus
D. Epstein–Barr virus
E. Rubella virus

148. Non-enveloped DNA viruses include:

A. Hepatitis B
B. Adenovirus
C. Papilloma
D. Mumps
E. Rotavirus

149. RNA viruses include:

A. Herpes simplex type 1
B. Rabies
C. Hepatitis A
D. Measles
E. Respiratory syncytial virus

150. *Escherichia coli*:

A. Is the most numerous commensal organism in the gut
B. Is nearly always sensitive to ampicillin
C. Is the most frequent aetiological agent in urinary tract infection
D. Produces bright pink colonies on MacConkey agar
E. Is an important cause of meningitis in neonates

151. The following are aminoglycoside antibiotics:

A. Amikacin
B. Streptomycin
C. Clindamycin
D. Gentamicin
E. Vancomycin

152. In pyogenic liver abscess:

A. Jaundice is a common presenting feature
B. *Staphylococcus aureus* is a common pathogen
C. Colonic pathology is often associated
D. Blood cultures are often positive
E. Prolonged antibiotics without drainage of pus is often curative

153. Infection with *Entamoeba histolytica*:

A. Usually affects the ileum
B. Is often asymptomatic
C. Is usually diagnosed by serological tests
D. Presents as a diffuse centrilobular necrosis when it affects the liver
E. Is treated with metronidazole

154. Impetigo in childhood:

A. Is due to streptococcal infection
B. May be associated with acute glomerulonephritis
C. Is a contagious disease
D. Usually presents as a rapidly-spreading erythematous rash
E. Is best treated with topical antibiotics

155. In the toxic shock syndrome:

A. The source of infection is usually contaminated tampons
B. The source of toxins is *Staphylococcus aureus*
C. Early antibiotic treatment leads to rapid resolution of symptoms
D. The rash is often vesicular
E. Phage typing is useful in confirming the diagnosis

156. Agents that interfere with viral multiplication include:

A. Amphotericin B
B. Amantadine
C. Metronidazole
D. Zidovudine
E. Ribavirin

157. The following may present as pyrexia of unknown origin:

A. Malaria
B. Toxoplasmosis
C. Pseudomembranous colitis
D. Brucellosis
E. Mumps

158. Adequate CSF levels of the following antimicrobial agents are achievable in bacterial meningitis:

A. Gentamicin
B. Ampicillin
C. Clarithromycin
D. Rifampicin
E. Chloramphenicol

159. Antigen detection in body fluids is useful in the diagnosis of infection due to:

A. Group B streptococci
B. *Haemophilus influenzae* type B
C. Coagulase-negative staphylococci
D. *Listeria monocytogenes*
E. *Streptococcus pneumoniae*

160. Varicella zoster virus (VZV):

A. Causes a vesicular rash
B. Grows quickly in tissue culture enabling early specific diagnosis
C. Is a cause of severe pneumonia
D. Is not sensitive to any available antiviral agents
E. Commonly causes latent infection

161. Typing of bacteria for epidemiological purposes can be done by the following methods:

A. Plasmid analysis
B. Antigenic profiling by serological methods
C. Bacteriophage typing
D. Gel electrophoresis of nucleic acid fragments produced by digestion with endonucleases
E. Antibiotic susceptibility patterns

162. Barrier nursing is used to prevent hospital cross-infection in the following:

A. Legionellosis
B. Malaria
C. Pseudomembranous colitis
D. Endocarditis
E. Typhoid fever

163. Trichomonas vaginalis:

A. Is sexually transmitted
B. May cause urethritis in males
C. Is easily diagnosed in 'wet' films of genital samples
D. Infection is treated with quinolones
E. May be found as a commensal in the gut

164. The following infections may be confirmed by examination of a Gram film of appropriate samples:

A. Whooping cough
B. Diphtheria
C. Gonococcal urethritis
D. Tuberculosis
E. Thrush

165. The following can be used for skin disinfection:

A. Quaternary ammonium compounds
B. Phenol
C. Glutaraldehyde
D. Alcoholic solution of chlorhexidine
E. Povidone–iodine solution

166. Airborne spread is important in:

A. Staphylococcal wound infection
B. Hepatitis E infection
C. Poliomyelitis
D. Campylobacter infection
E. Tuberculosis

167. Metronidazole is effective against:

A. *Giardia lamblia*
B. *Trichomonas vaginalis*
C. *Helicobacter pylori*
D. *Cryptosporidium* spp
E. *Bacteroides fragilis*

168. Respiratory syncytial virus (RSV):

A. Is not amenable to treatment with currently available antiviral agents
B. Causes bronchiolitis in infants
C. Does not produce lasting immunity
D. May cause severe illness in the elderly
E. Infection can be diagnosed rapidly by immunofluorescence

169. Causative agents of choroidoretinitis include:

A. Cytomegalovirus
B. Rubella
C. *Mycobacterium tuberculosis*
D. *Toxocara canis*
E. *Toxoplasma gondii*

170. Thick or thin blood films are useful in the diagnosis of:

A. Typhoid
B. Malaria
C. Filariasis
D. Trichomonas infection
E. Leprosy

171. Antifungal agents include:

A. Rifampicin
B. Amphotericin B
C. Flucytosine
D. Terbinafine
E. Ketoconazole

172. Cell-mediated immunity (type 4 hypersensitivity):

A. Evolves within 24 hours
B. Is important in controlling fungal diseases of the skin
C. Is responsible for a positive tuberculin skin test
D. Is diminished by treatment with steroids
E. Is characterised by a predominantly polymorphonuclear cell reaction locally after 48 hours

173. *Chlamydia trachomatis* is :

A. An obligate intracellular organism
B. The most common cause of sexually-transmitted disease in Western countries
C. The cause of lymphogranuloma venereum
D. Sensitive to erythromycin
E. A cause of community-acquired pneumonia

174. *Pasteurella multocida*:

A. Does not grow on routine bacterial culture media in the clinical laboratory
B. Is associated with animal bites
C. May cause rapidly-progressing cellulitis and septicaemia
D. Is sensitive to penicillin
E. Infection is prevented by immunisation which is recommended for veterinary workers

175. *Candida albicans*:

A. Can be differentiated from other *Candida* spp by its ability to form germ tubes
B. Is part of the normal flora of the gastrointestinal tract
C. Is a common cause of urinary tract infection
D. May cause infection of the mouth following the use of broad-spectrum antibiotics
E. Is sensitive to fluconazole

176. *Aspergillus* spp:

A. Are a rare but well-known cause of lung infection
B. Infection is often diagnosed by blood culture
C. Are often isolated from hospital air samples
D. May cause food poisoning
E. Are a common cause of superficial skin infections

177. The following can be detected by examination of a 'wet' film of urine:

A. White blood cells
B. Epithelial cells
C. *Mycobacterium* spp
D. Red blood cells
E. Bacteria

178. The following are common causes of urinary tract infection (UTI) in general practice:

A. *Enterococcus faecalis*
B. *Staphylococcus aureus*
C. *Proteus mirabilis*
D. *Escherichia coli*
E. *Klebsiella* spp

179. Bacterial ribosomes:

A. Can be visualised by light microscopy
B. Are associated with messenger RNA
C. Determine the sequence of amino acids in bacterial proteins
D. Are the site of action for aminoglycoside antibiotics
E. Are absent in obligate anaerobes

180. The cytoplasmic membrane:

A. Consists mainly of polysaccharides
B. Synthesis is prevented by β-lactam antibiotics
C. Contains endotoxin in Gram-negative bacteria
D. Is absent in *Mycoplasma* spp
E. Is a rigid structure in bacterial cells

Answers to Section III

121.
A – T Cryptosporidiosis is usually a self-limiting disease in normal people. However, in the severely immunocompromised, such as those with AIDS, it causes an intractable diarrhoea
B – T Person-to-person transmission may occur during outbreaks, particularly among young children
C – F Healthy children and adults are often infected, but infection is more severe in the immunocompromised
D – T Modified acid-fast stain is commonly used
E – T The organism is resistant to water chlorination

122.
A – T
B – F
C – F
D – T
E – F

123.
A – F
B – T
C – T
D – F
E – T
Other common causes of the common-cold syndrome are rhinoviruses and coronaviruses

124.
A – F *Bordetella pertussis* is isolated only from symptomatic patients
B – T
C – T
D – T
E – F

125.

A – F Maximal virus excretion and infectivity occurs in the early pre-icteric stage of the illness

B – F Chronic carriage does not occur with hepatitis A

C – T But person-to-person spread may occur where standards of hygiene are low

D – F But a recently introduced killed vaccine is available for persons at special risk

E – T Detection of IgM antibody provides relatively early diagnosis

126.

A – F

B – T

C – T

D – F

E – F

127.

A – T Part of the MMR (mumps, measles and rubella) vaccine is now routinely administered in childhood

B – T Though laboratory confirmation in typical cases is not necessary

C – T

D – T Other complications include orchitis, pancreatitis, meningo-encephalitis and, rarely, myocarditis

E – F Most commonly affects the parotid salivary glands

128.

A – T

B – F BCG is a live vaccine, an attenuated strain of bovine tuberculosis (Bacillus Calmette–Guérin)

C – F Aminoglycoside agents such as streptomycin are rarely used now, except for some resistant strains

D – F Infection with *Mycobacterium avium-intracellulare*, an atypical *Mycobacterium* species, is common in patients with AIDS, but the disease is not called tuberculosis

E – F Immunity is mainly cell-mediated

129.

A – T

B – T

C – T Hospital cross-infection has been shown in intensive care units and neonatal units

D – T Superficial *Candida* infections are common in AIDS

E – F

130.

A – F Staphylococci are common pathogens in cystic fibrosis, but not in chronic bronchitis

B – F *Streptococcus pneumoniae* is in fact a common cause

C – F Results of sputum culture are often difficult to interpret

D – T This is a useful objective indicator of bacterial infection

E – T

131.

A – F

B – T History of anaphylaxis after eating eggs

C – F The benefits of immunisation outweigh the risks of possible infection with the vaccine strain

D – F

E – F

132.

A – T

B – T

C – F The incubation period for hepatitis B infection is longer

D – T

E – T The vaccine consists of the surface antigen adsorbed onto aluminium hydroxide

133.

A – T Mediated by the epidermolytic toxin

B – F

C – T Mediated by the toxic shock syndrome toxin produced by some strains of *Staphylococcus aureus*

D – T

E – T Mediated by enterotoxins produced by some strains of *Staphylococcus aureus*

134.

A – F Typhoid fever itself is caused only by *Salmonella typhi*. Other 'enteric fevers' may be caused by species of *Salmonella* such as *S. paratyphi A* or *S. paratyphi B*

B – T

C – T The carrier state may be eradicated in some cases by prolonged treatment with agents such as ciprofloxacin

D – F Diagnosis is established by blood or stool culture

E – T This new vaccine, using the bio-engineered strain TY21a, is as effective as the killed parenteral vaccine

135.

A – F Hand, foot and mouth disease is caused by Coxsackie group A virus

B – T

C – T

D – F Cold sores are due to herpes simplex virus type I

E – F Vincent's angina is due to endogenous anaerobes such as *Borrelia vincenti* and *Fusobacterium* spp

136.

A – T

B – F Measles virus causes a macular rash

C – F As in B

D – T

E – F Rash is uncommon

137.

A – T

B – T

C – T

D – T

E – F

138.

A – T

B – F Listeriosis is an invasive infection

C – F

D – F This organism is not a cause of food poisoning

E – T Some strains of *Staphylococcus aureus* produce an enterotoxin

139.

A – F BCG is a live vaccine

B – F Whole cell vaccine is no longer used

C – T But a live oral vaccine is also now available

D – F Live vaccine is used, as part of MMR

E – F Formol toxoid is used for active immunisation

140.

A – F Type 1 hypersensitivity (anaphylaxis) is mediated by IgE antibodies

B – F

C – T

D – T

E – T

141.

A – F Antibiotic prophylaxis is needed only to cover procedures likely to be associated with transient bacteraemias, e.g. dental extraction

B – T To prevent recurrent group A streptococcal throat infection

C – T To reduce frequency and severity of recurrences

D – T To reduce likelihood of overwhelming sepsis with bacteria such as *Streptococcus pneumoniae, Streptococcus pyogenes* or *Neisseria meningitidis*

E – F Long-term antibiotic usage in this situation only leads to the emergence of resistant strains

142.

A – T

B – F The vast majority of strains are very sensitive to penicillin but resistant strains are emerging

C – T The vaccine contains the capsular polysaccharide from 23 of the more common serotypes of *Streptococcus pneumoniae*

D – F The typical appearance is of Gram-positive diplococci, i.e. in pairs

E – T

143.

A – T

B – F The coagulase test is an identification test for staphylococci (*Staphylococcus aureus* produces the enzyme coagulase)

C – T

D – T

E – F The polymerase chain reaction is used for the amplification and detection of small quantities of specific DNA

144.

A – T

B – F Needs to be used with caution, and only when there are no suitable alternatives

C – T Treatment of choice for amoebiasis, giardiasis and vaginal infections with *Trichomonas vaginalis*

D – T An alternative treatment is oral vancomycin

E – F

145.

A – T

B – T Cattle are a major reservoir of cryptosporidia

C – F But *Mycobacterium bovis*, now rare, can infect humans

D – T

E – T

146.

A – T This is particularly true in infants and in the elderly

B – T Toxin A and toxin B

C – F Toxins may occasionally be present in the stool sample in asymptomatic persons

D – T

E – T

147.

A – T

B – F

C – T

D – T

E – F

148.
A – ~~T~~ F
B – T
C – T
D – F
E – F

149.
A – F
B – T
C – T
D – T
E – T

150.
A – F By far the most numerous commensal organisms in the gut are anaerobes. *Escherichia coli* is the most numerous organism seen in aerobic cultures of stools
B – F 40–50% of strains are resistant to ampicillin
C – T
D – T i.e. it is a strong lactose fermenter
E – T *Escherichia coli* is an important cause of meningitis in the neonatal period

151.
A – T
B – T
C – F Clindamycin belongs to the macrolide group of antibiotics such as erythromycin
D – T
E – F Vancomycin is a cell-wall antibiotic useful for treating infection with resistant Gram-positive organisms such as methicillin-resistant staphylococci or enterococci

152.

A – F Jaundice is rarely a presenting feature in pyogenic liver abscess. The commonest presentation is as pyrexia of unknown origin (PUO)

B – F Infection is often due to multiple pathogens, commonly including *Streptococcus milleri*, coliform organisms and anaerobes. *Staphylococcus aureus* is uncommon

C – T Colonic pathology associated with pyogenic liver abscess includes diverticulosis, malignancy, Crohn's disease, ulcerative colitis and ischaemia

D – T Blood cultures are very useful in enabling isolation of pathogens

E – T Aspiration of pus is necessary only for diagnostic purposes in most cases

153.

A – F Usually affects the colon

B – T Particularly in endemic areas

C – F Serological tests are only useful in invasive disease such as liver abscess

D – F Liver involvement is always in the form of an abscess

E – T But to eliminate carriage of cysts, treatment with furamide (diloxanide furoate) is also necessary

154.

A – T But staphylococci may also be a cause

B – T

C – T

D – F Usually presents as a pustular rash

E – F Systemic antibiotics are advised

155.

A – T The causative organism (*Staphylococcus aureus*) is usually part of the endogenous flora of the patient. The tampon may be contaminated by the patient's fingers or from the perineum

B – T

C – F The effects of the toxin are not influenced by antibiotic treatment

D – F The rash is often erythematous and scaly

E – F Several phage types may be involved. Toxin testing is used to confirm aetiological agent

156.
A – F Amphotericin B is an antifungal agent
B – T Amantadine has useful activity against influenza A
C – F Metronidazole has antibacterial activity against anaerobic bacteria and certain protozoan pathogens such as *Entamoeba histolytica, Giardia lamblia* and *Trichomonas vaginalis*
D – T Zidovudine (AZT or azidothymidine) is active against HIV
E – T Ribavirin is active against the respiratory syncytial virus

157.
A – T
B – T
C – F
D – T
E – F Local signs and symptoms are pathognomonic

158.
A – F
B – T
C – F Macrolide antibiotics do not achieve sufficient concentrations in the CSF
D – T
E – T

159.
A – T
B – T
C – F
D – F
E – T

160.
A – T
B – F Diagnosis is established by serology
C – T Rare but well-recognised cause of serious pneumonia
D – F Is sensitive to acyclovir
E – T Reactivation of latent virus results in zoster

161.
A – T
B – T Useful for organisms such as *Salmonella* spp
C – T
D – T Variations based on this principle are now increasingly used for typing
E – T But this may not be sufficiently discriminatory

162.
A – F Person-to-person transmission has not been described
B – F
C – T
D – F
E – T

163.
A – T
B – T But the principal clinical manifestation is vaginitis
C – T
D – F Infection is treated with metronidazole
E – F But related species such as *Trichomonas hominis* may be found as commensals in the gut

164.
A – F Culture of pernasal swabs is needed
B – F Special stains such as Albert's stain is needed
C – T Presence of intracellular Gram-negative diplococci is diagnostic in gonococcal urethritis
D – F Acid-fast staining techniques such as Ziehl–Neelsen are necessary for diagnosis of tuberculosis
E – T *Candida albicans* stains as Gram-positive budding oval bodies

165.
A – F Quaternary ammonium compounds have only weak antiseptic activity
B – F Phenolics are too toxic for use on the skin
C – F As in B
D – T
E – T

166.
A – T
B – F Hepatitis E infection is spread by food or water
C – F As in B, but respiratory spread may also occur
D – F Usually a food-borne infection
E – T

167.
A – T
B – T
C – T Used in conjunction with another antibiotic such as amoxycillin or clarithromycin and a proton pump-inhibiting drug such as omeprezole for the treatment of *Helicobacter pylori* infection associated with gastric or duodenal ulcer
D – F There are no effective antibiotics for the treatment of *Cryptosporidium* infections
E – T *Bacteroides fragilis* is an obligate anaerobe commonly involved in anaerobic sepsis

168.
A – F Treatment with ribavirin is useful in severe cases
B – T
C – T Reinfection occurs commonly, even in the presence of antibody
D – T Severe illness in the elderly is not uncommon, particularly as outbreaks in nursing homes
E – T

169.
A – T Particularly in the immunocompromised
B – T Particularly as part of congenital rubella
C – T Tuberculous granulomas (nodules) in the retina are often seen in miliary tuberculosis
D – T
E – T Retinitis is one of the more serious manifestations of toxoplasmosis

170.

A – F Typhoid is diagnosed by isolation of the organism from stool culture or blood culture

B – T

C – T

D – F Trichomonas infection is diagnosed by examination of wet films of genital swabs

E – F Diagnosed by acid-fast staining of skin biopsies

171.

A – F Rifampicin is used mainly in treatment of tuberculosis

B – T

C – T

D – T Used mainly for treatment of fungal infections of nails

E – T

172.

A – F Usually take 48 hours or longer

B – T

C – T

D – T

E – F Cellular reaction locally is predominantly monocytic

173.

A – T

B – T Serotypes D through to K are involved

C – T Serotypes L1, L2 and L3 cause lymphogranuloma venereum

D – T Alternative therapy is tetracycline; newer macrolides such as clarithromycin or azithromycin may also be used.

E – F Acquired perinatally from infected mothers; the recently described species of *Chlamydia, C. pneumoniae*, is a common cause of pneumonia in adults

174.

A – F Grows easily on routine blood agar medium

B – T

C – T

D – T Quinolones such as ciprofloxacin are a good alternative

E – F No vaccine is available

175.

A – T

B – T But usually present in small numbers only

C – F Urinary tract infection is uncommon except in immuno-compromised patients or after catheterisation

D – T

E – T

176.

A – T Lung infection with *Aspergillus* spp, usually *Aspergillus fumigatus*, may present as allergic broncho-alveolar aspergillosis, invasive pulmonary aspergillosis or aspergilloma

B – F Blood culture is rarely positive

C – T *Aspergillus* spores are commonly found in the air

D – T Toxin production by *Aspergillus flavus* (aflatoxins) is responsible for this rare condition

E – F

177.

A – T

B – T

C – F Culture and identification tests are essential to identify *Mycobacterium* spp

D – T

E – T The presence of bacteria can be detected, though not their identity

178.

A – T

B – F *Staphylococcus aureus* is a rare cause of UTI

C – T Particularly in children

D – T *Escherichia coli* is the commonest cause

E – T

179.

A – F Can be visualised only by electron microscopy

B – T Are associated with messenger RNA in the cytoplasm to assemble proteins

C – F The sequence of amino acids is determined by the nuclear DNA, transcribed onto the messenger RNA

D – T

E – F All bacteria possess ribosomes

180.

A – F Consists mainly of lipoproteins

B – F β-lactam antibiotics such as penicillins and cephalosporins interfere with the synthesis of the cell wall, not the cytoplasmic membrane

C – F Endotoxin is part of the cell wall

D – F It is the cell wall which is absent in *Mycoplasma* spp

E – F

Section IV – Questions

181. Primary peritonitis:

A. Has a predilection for patients with ascites
B. Is often due to *Streptococcus pneumoniae*
C. Is more common than secondary peritonitis
D. Reveals foul-smelling pus upon laparotomy
E. Is an indication for treatment with penicillin

182. Antibiotic prophylaxis for colonic surgery:

A. Has been shown to be of clear benefit
B. Should ideally be started 3 days before surgery
C. Should always include metronidazole
D. Depends on achieving adequate levels of antibiotics in the bowel lumen
E. Is directed mainly at the prevention of tetanus and gas gangrene

183. Adverse reactions to oral penicillin include:

A. Convulsions
B. Cholestatic jaundice
C. Type 1 hypersensitivity (anaphylaxis)
D. Diarrhoea
E. Macular rash if taken when suffering from infectious mononucleosis

184. Monitoring of blood levels of the antibiotic is routinely indicated during treatment with:

A. Cephalosporins
B. Vancomycin
C. Rifampicin
D. Gentamicin
E. Acyclovir

185. *Klebsiella pneumoniae*:

A. Is a common cause of lobar pneumonia
B. Is usually sensitive to ampicillin
C. Is a capsulate organism
D. Often forms part of the commensal flora of the gut
E. Causes nosocomial (hospital-acquired) urinary tract infections

186. Lung abscess:

A. May occur as a complication of pneumococcal lobar pneumonia
B. Often requires surgical drainage in addition to antibiotics
C. When multiple, usually indicates staphylococcal sepsis
D. Often requires multiple (combined) antibiotic therapy
E. Is more common in patients with chronic bronchitis (chronic obstructive alveolar disease)

187. Sore throat with fever:

A. Is due to *Streptococcus pyogenes* in most cases
B. Should always be treated with penicillin or erythromycin
C. When recurrent is an indication for tonsillectomy
D. May be rapidly diagnosed by detection of raised anti-streptolysin O titre in the serum
E. Is classically associated with acute glomerulonephritis

188. Cholangitis:

A. May occur as a complication of hepatitis A infection
B. Is commonly due to coliform organisms
C. Often leads to septicaemia and positive blood culture
D. Is adequately treated with ampicillin
E. May lead to multiple abscess formation in the liver

189. Rifampicin is useful in the management of the following conditions:

A. Pneumococcal meningitis
B. Tuberculous meningitis
C. Meningococcal meningitis
D. Legionnaires' disease
E. Infections caused by methicillin-resistant *Staphylococcus aureus* (MRSA)

190. Leishmaniasis:

A. Has been eradicated in Europe
B. Is spread by mosquitoes
C. Is usually diagnosed by examination of stained films of peripheral blood
D. Commonly presents as cutaneous leishmaniasis in the middle-eastern countries
E. Is effectively treated with chloroquine

191. Antibiotics appropriate for 'blind' therapy of urinary tract infections in general practice include:

A. Trimethoprim
B. Erythromycin
C. Co-amoxiclav (augmentin)
D. Oral cephalosporins
E. Chloramphenicol

192. In mycobacterial infection of the genito-urinary tract:

A. The renal pelvis is most commonly affected
B. Nephrectomy is usually necessary in addition to antituberculous chemotherapy
C. Positive microscopy for acid-fast bacilli in an early morning sample of urine is usually diagnostic
D. Sterile pyuria on routine urine culture is a consistent finding
E. *Mycobacterium tuberculosis* is the species most commonly involved

193. The following roundworms may cause infections in man:

A. *Strongyloides stercoralis*
B. *Taenia saginata*
C. *Paragonimus westermanii*
D. *Trichuris trichiura*
E. *Enterobius vermicularis*

194. *Neisseria gonorrhoeae*:

A. Is a Gram-negative diplococcus
B. Is reliably sensitive to penicillin
C. May cause systemic infection
D. Infection in females usually presents with purulent vaginal discharge
E. Can be serotyped for epidemiological purposes

195. Treatment with acyclovir:

A. Is effective in infections with varicella-zoster virus
B. If started early results in eradication of infection
C. Is contra-indicated in pregnancy
D. Selectively inhibits viral DNA-polymerase activity in infected cells
E. Is frequently associated with hypersensitivity reactions

196. Pathogens that are transmitted by penetrating injury with blood-contaminated sharps include:

A. Epstein–Barr virus
B. Hepatitis A virus
C. Hepatitis C virus
D. *Plasmodium falciparum*
E. HIV

197. Cavitating lesions are a feature of pulmonary infections with:

A. *Aspergillus* spp
B. *Mycoplasma pneumoniae*
C. *Haemophilus influenzae*
D. *Nocardia* spp
E. *Klebsiella pneumoniae*

198. Organisms associated with intra-cerebral abscesses include:

A. *Neisseria meningitidis*
B. *Entamoeba histolytica*
C. *Streptococcus milleri*
D. *Peptostreptococcus anaerobius*
E. *Actinomyces israelii*

199. Organisms associated with acute infective colitis include:

A. Rotavirus
B. *Salmonella typhi*
C. *Clostridium difficile*
D. *Shigella dysenteriae*
E. *Entamoeba coli*

200. Enteric fever may be caused by:

A. *Enterococcus faecalis*
B. *Salmonella typhi*
C. *Giardia lamblia*
D. *Salmonella paratyphi A*
E. *Salmonella enteritidis*

201. Ringworm infections:

A. Are diseases of the stratum corneum of the skin
B. May be associated with *Trichophyton rubrum*
C. Can be caused by *Microsporum canis*
D. Are spread by contact with an infected individual or animal
E. Induce development of active T cell-mediated immunity

202. In HIV infection:

A. Monitoring of the number of T4 cells (CD4 cells) is a useful guide to the onset of AIDS
B. Numbers of T8 cells (CD8 cells) increase as disease develops
C. The virus is found in monocyte-macrophage cells
D. The HIV virus is not present in plasma
E. Prolonged treatment with combined antiviral agents is curative

203. HIV is reliably inactivated by:

A. The autoclave
B. The hot-air oven
C. Chlorhexidine
D. Glutaraldehyde
E. Hypochlorites

204. Acute and convalescent sera are required to make a definitive serological diagnosis of infection because:

A. Non-specific antibodies may be present in the first serum
B. One serum may not possess sufficient complement
C. High levels of antibody must be demonstrated in both sera
D. A rising antibody titre is significant
E. One serum may contain an antibiotic

205. Cephalosporins effective when given orally are

A. Ceftazidime
B. Cephalexin
C. Cefuroxime
D. Cefaclor
E. Cefotaxime

206. Antimicrobial agents with a good spectrum of activity against anaerobic bacteria include

A. Vancomycin
B. Chloramphenicol
C. Co-amoxyclav
D. Clindamycin
E. Gentamicin

207. Are the following statements true or false?

A. Transplacental transfer of antibody results in natural active immunity in the foetus
B. Administration of toxoid results in artificial active immunity
C. Administration of antitoxin results in artificial passive immunity
D. Subclinical infection results in natural passive immunity
E. Administration of γ-globulin results in artificial passive immunity

208. *Streptococcus pyogenes*:

A. Can be isolated from the throat swab of some 'normal' individuals
B. Is a facultative anaerobe
C. Is a common urinary tract pathogen
D. May develop resistance to penicillin during prolonged treatment
E. Infections are often treated with aminoglycosides

209. Phage typing is used in epidemiological studies to discriminate among:

A. *Staphylococcus aureus*
B. *Streptococcus pneumoniae*
C. *Salmonella enteritidis*
D. *Mycobacterium tuberculosis*
E. *Neisseria gonorrhoeae*

210. Factors affecting the performance of a disinfectant are:

A. pH
B. Temperature
C. Number of organisms present
D. Concentration of disinfectant
E. Type of organisms

211. Bacterial spores:

A. Are killed by a temperature of 120°C for 20 minutes
B. Can be stained by Gram's method
C. Multiply in adverse environments
D. Are resistant to antibiotics
E. Are formed only by Gram-positive bacilli

212. DNA may be transferred naturally among bacteria by:

A. Recombination
B. Transduction
C. Conjugation
D. Transcription
E. Mutation

213. Bacterial plasmids:

A. Are extrachromosomal genetic elements
B. May code for virulence factors
C. Can be separated by electrophoretic techniques
D. May be transmissible amongst different species of bacteria
E. May be used to characterise bacterial strains

214. Yellow fever is endemic in:

A. The Caribbean
B. China
C. Nigeria
D. Brazil
E. India

215. The following are human herpes viruses:

A. Epstein–Barr virus
B. Cytomegalovirus
C. Varicella-zoster virus
D. Rabies virus
E. ECHO virus

216. Bacteria that may cause infections characterised by skin rash include:

A. *Borrelia burgdorferi*
B. *Salmonella typhi*
C. Group A streptococcus
D. *Streptococcus pneumoniae*
E. *Neisseria gonorrhoeae*

217. Slaughterhouse workers have a higher than average likelihood of infection with the following:

A. *Coxiella burneti*
B. *Salmonella typhi*
C. *Brucella* spp
D. *Leptospira* spp
E. *Streptococcus suis*

218. *Cryptococcus neoformans*:

A. Is a yeast
B. Capsular antigens can be detected in serum and cerebrospinal fluid in cases of meningitis
C. May cause pneumonia
D. Is sensitive to amphotericin B
E. Is found in bird, particularly pigeon, droppings

219. *Giardia lamblia* infection:

A. May be diagnosed by serological tests
B. Is caused by ingestion of cysts
C. May be spread as a zoonosis
D. Affects mainly the ileocaecal region
E. May cause a malabsorption syndrome

220. Medically-important protozoa include:

A. *Leishmania donovani*
B. *Schistosoma mansonii*
C. *Trypanosoma cruzei*
D. *Echinococcus granulosus*
E. *Toxoplasma gondii*

221. Infection with *Vibrio cholerae*:

A. Is best prevented by vaccination
B. Produces severe inflammation of the small bowel
C. Is effectively treated with oral or parenteral antibiotics
D. Is transmitted with drinking water and food
E. May be spread as a zoonosis

222. *Helicobacter pylori*:

A. Rarely infects people in developed countries
B. Is transmitted with food or drinking water
C. May be identified by its production of urease
D. Infection may be diagnosed by a serological test
E. Infection can be eradicated by antibiotic therapy

223. Mycobacterium avium-intracellulare:

A. Is a member of the *Mycobacterium tuberculosis* complex
B. Causes cervical lymphadenopathy in children
C. Causes disseminated infections in the elderly
D. Produces relatively rapidly-growing colonies on culture
E. Is a common opportunistic bacterial pathogen in patients with AIDS

224. Organisms associated with atypical pneumonia are:

A. *Streptococcus pneumoniae*
B. *Chlamydia psittaci*
C. *Mycoplasma hominis*
D. *Chlamydia pneumoniae*
E. *Influenza viruses*

225. In a young adult presenting with acute meningitis:

A. Treatment should be delayed until a CSF sample is obtained so that an aetiological diagnosis can be established
B. Blood cultures are unlikely to be helpful
C. Antigen detection tests may be positive even after antibiotic treatment
D. A predominantly lymphocytic CSF cell-count excludes bacterial meningitis
E. Erythromycin is the drug of choice in patients who are allergic to penicillin

226. Infection of closed CSF shunts installed for the relief of hydrocephalus:

A. Presents with swinging pyrexia
B. Is mostly due to skin organisms such as *Staphylococcus epidermidis* or diphtheroids
C. May be diagnosed by positive blood cultures
D. Results in nephritis due to haematogenous spread of infection to the kidneys
E. Can often be successfully eradicated with intra-ventricular administration of antibiotics

227. In anaerobic vaginosis:

A. Numerous pus cells are seen on microscopy
B. Culture often yields *Gardnerella vaginalis*
C. Symptoms are relieved by measures to reduce the acidity of the vaginal secretions
D. Treatment with metronidazole is effective
E. Infection is often sexually-transmitted

228. Bacteria commonly causing sepsis in burns include:

A. *Streptococcus pyogenes*
B. *Clostridium perfringens*
C. *Staphylococcus aureus*
D. *Bacteroides melaninogenicus*
E. *Pseudomonas aeruginosa*

229. Plantar warts:

A. Are caused by papillomaviruses
B. Are due to infection of subcutaneous cells in the soles of the feet
C. Elicit strong cell-mediated immunity
D. May lead to epithelial neoplasms
E. Are caused by a virus which can be grown on epithelial cell cultures

230. Scabies:

A. Mainly affects immunocompromised patients
B. Is caused by infection of the superficial layers of the skin with *Sarcoptes scabei*
C. Has been eradicated in developed countries
D. Presents as an itchy rash mainly affecting the trunk
E. Is diagnosed by microscopic examination of skin swabs

231. *Streptococcus pneumoniae* is associated with:

A. Pyogenic arthritis
B. Brain abscess
C. Primary peritonitis
D. Empyema
E. Pyelonephritis

232. Viruses associated with conjunctivitis include:

A. Herpes simplex
B. Adenovirus
C. Varicella-zoster
D. Rubella
E. Influenza A

233. β-lactam-derived antibiotics with activity against *Pseudomonas* spp include:

A. Meropenem
B. Flucloxacillin
C. Cefuroxime
D. Ceftazidime
E. Ciprofloxacin

234. The following is/are true of tuberculosis:

A. The majority of new cases in the UK are among immigrants
B. Immunity is mainly cell-mediated
C. Subclinical infection in childhood leaves long-lasting immunity
D. In pulmonary disease the lung bases are most often affected
E. Laboratory culture and sensitivity tests may take several weeks to complete

235. Diseases associated with *Clostridium perfringens* include:

A. Pseudomembranous colitis
B. Necrotising enterocolitis
C. Gas gangrene
D. Food poisoning
E. Necrotising fasciitis

236. Direct immunofluorescence tests on sputum smears are helpful in the rapid diagnosis of infections with:

A. *Legionella pneumophila*
B. *Mycobacterium tuberculosis*
C. Respiratory syncytial virus
D. *Pneumocystis carinii*
E. *Bordetella pertussis*

237. Urinary tract infection in pregnancy:

A. Needs to be treated even if asymptomatic
B. May be treated with quinolone antibiotics
C. Is often due to uncommon organisms such as *Pseudomonas* spp
D. Is more likely to include pyelonephritis
E. Is more likely to relapse after treatment

238. The following antimicrobial agents are rapidly absorbed and systemically effective after oral administration:

A. Metronidazole
B. Vancomycin
C. Acyclovir
D. Fusidic acid
E. Amphotericin B

239. Infections due to *Shigella* spp:

A. Are usually seen only among returning travellers and recent immigrants to the UK
B. Often present clinically as severe watery diarrhoea
C. Often produce positive blood cultures
D. Are not preventable by vaccination
E. May require antibiotic therapy in severe cases

240. Pathogens which cause cervical lymphadenopathy in children include:

A. *Mycobacterium avium-intracellulare*
B. Rubella virus
C. *Streptococcus pyogenes*
D. Mumps virus
E. *Haemophilus influenzae* type B

Answers to Section IV

181.
A – T Patients with renal failure and young girls are other groups at risk
B – T *Streptococcus pneumoniae* is the commonest cause, followed by *Streptococcus pyogenes*
C – F Primary peritonitis is an uncommon condition
D – F The pus in primary peritonitis is not foul-smelling, in contrast to peritonitis following perforation of the bowel. The latter is associated with anaerobes from the colon
E – T

182.
A – T
B – F Should ideally be started with induction of anaesthesia
C – T
D – F Depends on achieving adequate levels of antibiotics in the tissues
E – F Is directed mainly at the prevention of infection by non-sporing anaerobes and coliforms

183.
A – T May occur with high doses especially in renal failure
B – F
C – T This is the commonest serious side effect
D – T
E – F But this is a consistent phenomenon with ampicillin/amoxycillin

184.
A – F
B – T
C – F But measurement may occasionally be required if there is uncertainty about absorption during oral therapy
D – T
E – F

185.

A – F   *Klebsiella* spp are a rare cause of lobar pneumonia
B – F   Always resistant to ampicillin
C – T
D – T   But present only in small numbers
E – T   Particularly in patients with indwelling catheters

186.

A – F
B – F   Prolonged antibiotic therapy alone is usually sufficient
C – T   Right-sided endocarditis or osteomyelitis is often the source
D – T   Since more than one organism (including anaerobes) may be involved, especially if secondary to aspiration
E – F

187.

A – F   Half or more cases are due to viral infection
B – F   In many cases treatment may be deferred until results of tests for streptococcal infection are available
C – T
D – F   Rise in antibody titre may not occur for 2 weeks or more
E – F   Streptococcal sore throat is classically associated with rheumatic fever. Acute glomerulonephritis is also associated with streptococcal impetigo

188.

A – F
B – T
C – T
D – F   The organisms involved are frequently resistant to ampicillin
E – T

189.

A – F
B – T   As part of combination therapy with other anti-tuberculous agents such as isoniazid, ethambutol and pyrazinamide
C – T   For elimination of carriage of meningococci
D – T   In combination with erythromycin
E – T   Usually in combination with another agent such as fusidic acid

190.

A – F Endemic in southern Europe
B – F Spread by sandflies
C – F Usually diagnosed by examination of bone marrow or splenic aspirate
D – T
E – F Treatment is with antimonial compounds for visceral leishmaniasis

191.

A – T
B – F Most urinary pathogens are resistant to erythromycin
C – T
D – T
E – F The incidence of serious side effects with chloramphenicol is too high to allow its use in a common condition such as UTI

192.

A – T
B – F Antituberculous chemotherapy alone is sufficient in nearly all cases
C – F Acid-fast bacilli seen in samples of urine often turn out to be contaminating atypical mycobacteria when culture and identification are completed
D – T Sterile pyuria refers to absence of bacterial growth on routine culture of a sample of urine with numerous pus cells
E – T

193.

A – T
B – F *Taenia saginata* is a flat worm (cestode)
C – F *Paragonimus westermanii* is the lung fluke (trematode)
D – T
E – T

194.

A – T
B – F Many strains are now resistant
C – T Disseminated gonococcal infection is a rare but well-known and serious condition
D – F Infection in females is often minimally symptomatic
E – T

195.
A – T
B – F Infection is only suppressed, and remains latent
C – F May be used with caution in pregnancy
D – T
E – F Hypersensitivity reactions are rare

196.
A – F
B – F
C – T
D – F
E – T

197.
A – T
B – F
C – F
D – T
E – T Often as part of aspiration pneumonia

198.
A – F
B – T Brain abscesses are a rare but well-known complication of amoebiasis
C – T *Streptococcus milleri* is one of the more common causes of pyogenic brain abscess. It is often associated with anaerobes
D – T See also C
E – T Metastatic infection in the brain occasionally occurs in actinomycosis

199.
A – F Predominantly affects the small bowel
B – F As in A
C – T
D – T
E – T

200.
A – F
B – T
C – F
D – T
E – F

The term 'enteric fever' refers to the syndrome of prolonged, systemic pyrexial illness due to certain invasive species of *Salmonella*, i.e. *S. typhi* and *S. paratyphi A, B* and *C*. Rarely, other species of *Salmonella* such as *S. virchow* may also produce a similar clinical syndrome

201.
A – T
B – T
C – T   *Microsporum canis* infection is usually acquired from pets
D – T
E – T

202.
A – T   CD4 cell counts of less than $200/mm^3$ portend the onset of AIDS
B – F   Though CD8 cells initially increase in numbers relative to CD4 cells, all lymphocytes decrease in numbers as disease progresses
C – T   Though infected, these cells are less easily killed by the virus
D – F
E – F   Combination treatment with agents such as zidovudine (AZT), didanosine(DDI) and zalcitabine (DDC), will delay progress of the disease, but does not eradicate infection

203.
A – T
B – T
C – F   Chlorhexidine is effective but does not guarantee complete elimination of HIV
D – T
E – T

204.
A – F
B – F
C – F
D – T
E – F

205.
A – F
B – T
C – T   As the ester, cefuroxime axetil
D – T
E – F

206.
A. T   Active against Gram-positive anaerobes only.
B. T   But seldom used because of potential toxicity
C. T   But metronidazole is preferred in serious anaerobic infections
D. T
E. F   Aminoglycoside antibiotics are ineffective against anaerobes

207.
A – F   This represents natural passive immunity
B – T
C – T
D – F   This represents natural active immunity
E – T

208.
A – T
B – T   I.e. it grows both aerobically and anaerobically
C – F   Urinary tract infection with this pathogen is very rare
D – F   Resistance to penicillin is unknown
E – F   This organism is always resistant to aminoglycosides

209.
A – T
B – F   Distinguished by serotyping
C – T
D – F   Though possible, phage typing is rarely used
E – F   As in B

210.

A – T

B – T

C – T

D – T

E – T

211.

A – T

B – F   Spores are not stained by Gram's method

C – F   Spores stay dormant during adverse conditions

D – T   Antibiotics act by interfering with bacterial metabolic pathways and so cannot affect the dormant spores

E – T   Are formed mainly by Gram-positive genera such as *Clostridium* and *Bacillus*

212.

A – F   True recombination only occurs during meiosis in diploid cells

B – T   Refers to transfer of DNA via non-lethal viruses which infect bacteria (bacteriophages)

C – T   Refers to mating and direct transfer of DNA between bacterial cells in contact

D – F   Refers to copying of information from DNA to mRNA

E – F   Refers to heritable changes in the nucleotide sequence of DNA

213.

A – T

B – T   May code for virulence factors such as toxin production

C – T

D – T   May be transmissible between related species

E – T   Plasmid profiles may be used to characterise bacterial strains

214.

A – T

B – F

C – T   And in most of equatorial Africa

D – T   And in most of South America

E – F

215.
A – T
B – T
C – T
D – F Rabies virus belongs to the rhabdoviridae
E – F ECHO virus is an enterovirus

216.
A – T *Borrelia burgdorferi* infection is characterised by erythema chronicum migrans at the site of the tick bite
B – T *Salmonella typhi* infection produces the characteristic rose spots
C – T Group A streptococcus infection may be complicated by scarlet fever
D – F
E – T Disseminated gonococcal infection produces a pustular rash

217.
A – T
B – F
C – T
D – T Caused by *Leptospira hebdomidis*
E – T *Streptococcus suis* is a pathogen found in the nasopharynx of pigs. It causes meningo-encephalitis following accidental inoculation

218.
A – T A capsulate yeast. Non-capsulate variants occur
B – T
C – T Pneumonia and invasion of the bloodstream may occur in the immunocompromised
D – T Amphotericin B is often used in combination with 5-flucytosine
E – T

219.
A – F Diagnosis is by microscopy of stool samples or jejunal aspirates
B – T Cysts are found in contaminated water supplies
C – T Many mammals, especially rodents, are infected with *Giardia* spp, which may occasionally be transmitted to man
D – F Affects mainly the duodenum and jejunum
E – T

220.
A – T
B – F
C – T
D – F
E – T

221.
A – F Vaccination against cholera is of poor efficacy; prevention is by ensuring a clean water supply and good food hygiene
B – F Inflammatory changes are minimal
C – F The mainstay of treatment is oral or parenteral rehydration
D – T
E – F Infection only involves humans

222.
A – F But infection is more prevalent in older age groups in developed countries
B – F Infection is transmitted from person to person
C – T
D – T
E – T Combination therapy with a proton-pump inhibitor and two antibiotics for one week is usually effective

223.
A – F Members of the *Mycobacterium tuberculosis* complex include *M. tuberculosis, M. bovis, M. africanum* and *M. microti*
B – T It is the commonest cause of cervical lymphadenopathy in children in western countries
C – F Causes disseminated infections only in severely immunocompromised patients
D – F Produces non-pigmented, slow-growing colonies
E – T

224.
A – F Pneumococcal pneumonia is not classified as an 'atypical pneumonia'
B – T
C – F *Mycoplasma pneumoniae* is a common cause, not *M. hominis*
D – T
E – T

225.

A – F Antibiotics should be started without delay, after obtaining blood culture if possible. Antigen testing in serum, urine or CSF may allow the aetiology to be established even after antibiotics have been started and cultures are negative

B – F Blood cultures are often positive

C – T

D – F A lymphocytic CSF may be found in partially-treated pyogenic meningitis and in tuberculous meningitis

E – F Erythromycin does not cross the blood–CSF barrier

226.

A – F Presents with low-grade pyrexia

B – T

C – T

D – F Nephritis does occur, but is immune complex-mediated

E – F Attempts at eradication with antibiotics are often unsuccessful

227.

A – F Pus cells are 'remarkable by their absence'

B – T Other organisms seen include *Mobiluncus* spp and anaerobes

C – F Anaerobic vaginosis is characterised by high (alkaline) pH. Topical gels containing low pH buffers may help when the standard treatment, metronidazole, cannot be used

D – T

E – F There is no good evidence for this

228.

A – T

B – F

C – T

D – F

E – T

229.

A – T But the organism has not been grown on tissue culture

B – F Infection affects the stratum corneum

C – F The immune response is often ineffective

D – F Though some members of this family of viruses are associated with neoplasms, plantar or common skin warts are not

E – F

230.

A – F May affect individuals with normal immune function, but a severe form may occur in the immunocompromised (Norwegian scabies)

B – T

C – F Is still prevalent where standards of personal hygiene are low

D – F The itchy rash mainly affects the flexor aspects of the joints and areas with loose skin folds

E – F Diagnosed by microscopic examination of scrapings obtained from the burrows in the skin

231.

A – T

B – T Often secondary to sinusitis or otitis media

C – T

D – T Often secondary to lobar pneumonia

E – F

232.

A – T

B – T

C – T As part of ophthalmic zoster

D – F Congenital rubella causes choroidoretinitis, not conjunctivitis

E – F

233.

A – T

B – F Flucloxacillin has activity only against Gram-positive organisms

C – F

D – T

E – F Ciprofloxacin does have good activity against *Pseudomonas* spp, but it is not a β-lactam antibiotic

234.

A – F Though the incidence is relatively high among recent immigrants, especially in London, the majority of UK cases occur in the native population

B – T

C – F Infection often remains dormant and may become active in later life

D – F The apical lobe is most often affected

E – T

235.

A – F Pseudomembranous colitis is caused by toxigenic strains of *Clostridium difficile*

B – T

C – T

D – T

E – F Necrotising fasciitis is caused most commonly by *Streptococcus pyogenes*, though other organisms may also be involved

236.

A – T

B – F The fluorescent auramine-phenol stain is often used but is not a specific immunological stain

C – T

D – T

E – F

237.

A – T

B – F Quinolone antibiotics (nalidixic acid, norfloxacin, ciprofloxacin, etc) are best avoided in pregnancy

C – F The pathogens involved are mostly the usual agents causing UTI such as *Escherichia coli*, *Proteus mirabilis*, other coliforms, entero-cocci, coagulase-negative staphylococci, etc

D – T

E – T

238.

A – T

B – F The oral preparation is intended to be active only in the gut lumen

C – T

D – T

E – F As in B

239.

A – F Shigellosis, particularly that due to *Shigella sonnei*, is endemic in many developed countries

B – F The usual presenting symptom is frequent small stools with blood and mucus

C – F Blood culture is rarely positive

D – T

E – T Quinolone antibiotics are recommended in severe cases

240.

A – T

B – T

C – T

D – F

E – F